WHAT IN THE WORLD IS
RH DISEASE?

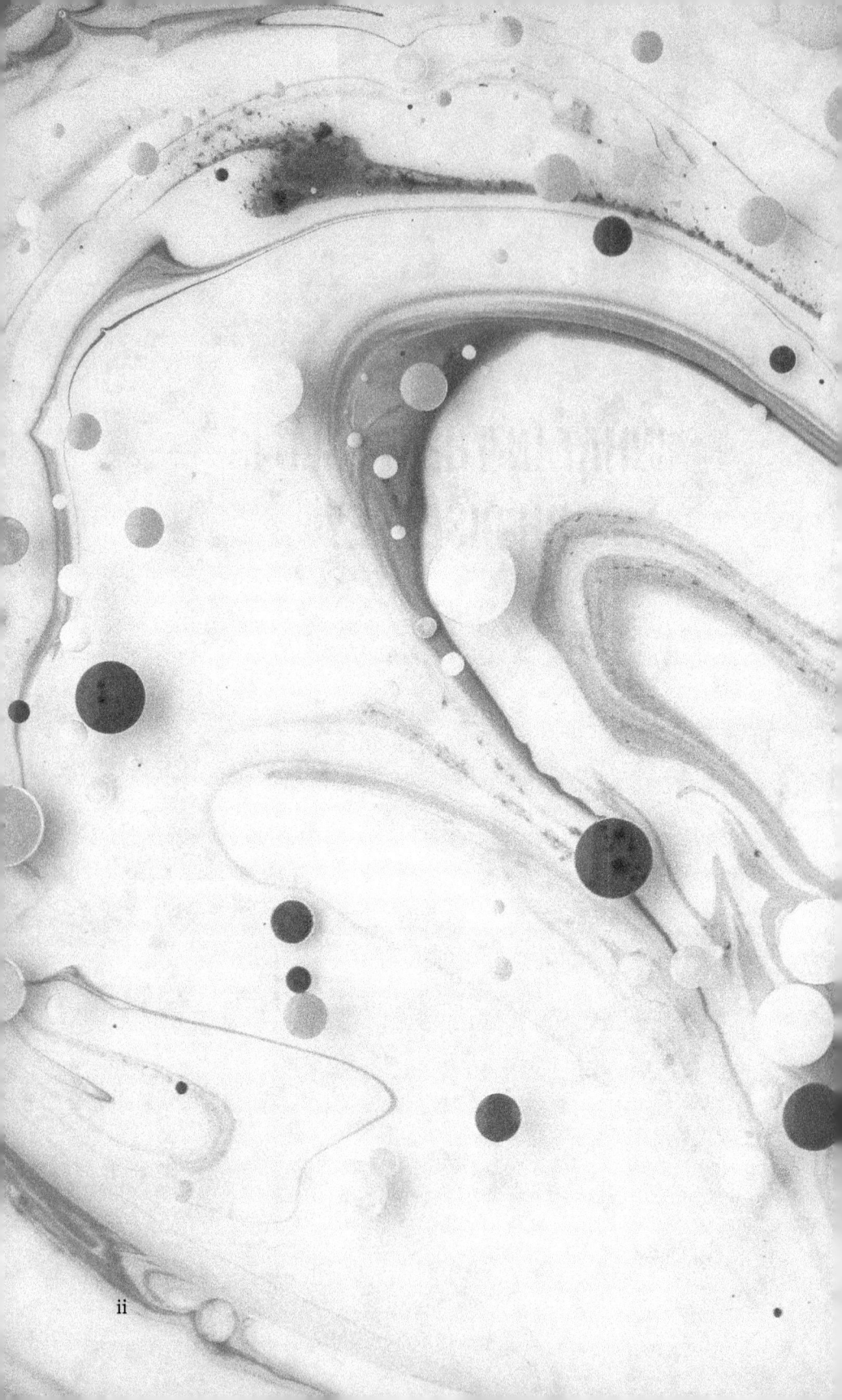

ii

WHAT IN THE WORLD IS RH DISEASE?

Dr. Austin Mardon, Sheher-Bano Ahmed,
Joonsoo Sean Lyeo, Rodala Aranya, Pareesa Ali,
Dhwani Bhadresa, Samira Sunderji, Si Cong (Sam) Zhang,
Anusha Mappanasingam, Rishi Thangarajah,
Salma Abrahim, Rahma Gulaid, Olivia Brodowski

2021

First Printing: 2021

Typeset and Cover Design by Anna Kraemer

ISBN 978-1-77369-239-5

Golden Meteorite Press
103 11919 82 St NW
Edmonton, AB T5B 2W3
www.goldenmeteoritepress.com

CONTENTS

INTRODUCTION

T HIS BOOK WAS CREATED through the Antarctic Institute of Canada as a project sponsored by the Government of Canada's innovative Work-Integrated Learning program, Level Up. The Antarctic Institute of Canada is a non-profit Canadian charity organization founded in 1985 by former Antarctic researcher Austin Mardon. Its original aim was to lobby for the federal government of Canada to increase the extent of Canadian research in the Antarctic. Today, its objectives also include supporting scholarly research and academic writing.

A group of twelve postsecondary students worked on this book over a period of seven days. Each chapter was written by a different student, with some chapters being created through the collaborative efforts of multiple authors. All editing, graphic design, and audiobook production was also carried out by postsecondary students.

In creating this book, we hope to provide information on Rh disease and perhaps help eradicate it for good. Too often, information about medical disorders is hidden behind technical jargon or is frustratingly vague and confusing.

With this book, we hope to introduce readers to Rh disease in a way that is both comprehensive and easy to understand. We hope that our readers will find this book useful for understanding both the medical aspects of Rh disease as well as its societal impacts. Thank you for taking the time to learn more about this disease.

CHAPTER 1

What Did People Think RH Disease was Before its Discovery?

Written By Joonsoo Sean Lyeo

RHESUS (RH) DISEASE occurs when the antibodies present in a pregnant woman's blood cross the placental barrier and damage the unborn baby's red blood cells (Clarke, 1967). Nowadays, this phenomenon is fairly well-understood in academic circles. It is currently known that Rh disease occurs as the result of a mother with Rh negative blood, whose immune system has previously been exposed or sensitized to Rh positive blood, carrying a baby with Rh positive blood. The condition can be fatal if left undiagnosed, but modern interventions allow for the early detection and prevention of Rh blood incompatibility (Costumbrado, Mansour, & Ghassemzadeh, 2020). As a result of these innovations, the prevalence of Rh disease has dropped to less than 3 cases for every 100,000 live births in developed countries (Costumbrado, Mansour, & Ghassemzadeh, 2020).

That being said, the scientific community was not always privy to the knowledge underlying Rh disease and how it manifests. It wasn't until 1939, less than a century ago, when physicians Dr. Philip Levine and Dr. Rufus E. Stetson were able to identify an association between the death of a stillborn baby and the Rh blood incompatibility of their parents (Levine & Stetson, 1939). The pair described the account of a woman who had received three blood transfusions from her husband following a period of considerable blood loss (Levine & Stetson, 1939). While their blood should've been compatible, based on the prevailing understanding of the ABO system, the woman experienced a severe reaction to her husband's blood. From this observation, the authors correctly suggested that there must be some human blood antigen, which had not been accounted for by the ABO system, causing this unexpected blood incompatibility (Stockman Iii, 2001). This observation predicated the eventual discovery of the Rh antigen, carried by only a relatively slim minority of the total human population. For more information on how this crucial discovery contributed to the study of hemolytic disease, please refer to "Chapter 3: How Did the Discovery of RH Disease Impact the Study of Hemolytic Diseases?"

Prior to this discovery, as well as the subsequent innovations in treatment methods and tools, the condition now known as Rh disease became a leading cause of perinatal death (Queenan, 2002). It should be noted that the term 'perinatal death' refers to the death of a child either while they are still in the womb, or shortly after their time of birth (Queenan, 2002). At the time of this discovery, an estimated half of all women with Rh negative blood, specifically those who had previously been sensitized to Rh positive blood through injury or prior pregnancy, were at risk of losing their baby either in the womb or shortly after birth (Queenan, 2002).

Suffice to say, ignorance was not bliss. Long before it received its current name, or before its underlying mechanism was fully understood, Rh disease was understood to have been a major cause of fetal and neonatal death. Some investigators have argued that the earliest recorded descriptions of Rh disease, and the perinatal deaths caused by this affliction, date back to the works of Hippocrates in 400 BC (Jackson & Baker, 2021). These medical historians contend that Hippocrates' description of a condition, which he termed 'fetus carnosus', bore a strong resemblance to modern depictions of Rh disease. In his description of fetus carnosus, as seen in a case study provided in *The Epidemics*, Hippocrates described the birth of a 'fleshy fetus' with 'general fetal dropsy' (Baskett, 2019).

While other records seemingly matching the symptoms of Rh disease surfaced in the interim, former Duke University professor Dr. Wendell Franklyn Rosse argued that the most notable, and perhaps the most historically significant, examples of perinatal death caused by Rh disease occurred nearly two millennia later (Rosse, 1990). In 1509, Catherine of Aragon married King Henry the VIII of England and, over the course of the next 19 years, bore him six children (Stockman Iii, 2001). Of these six children, five died in utero or early infancy. As an aside, the sole surviving daughter was Mary Tudor, who eventually succeeded her father as Queen of England (Stockman Iii, 2001).

At the time, several hypotheses were put forward to explain the possible cause of Catherine's series of miscarriages. Believing the marriage was cursed, Henry himself turned to the biblical *Book of Leviticus*, in which he cited the verses 18:16 and 20:21 as evidence that his infertility woes were the result of divine punishment for marrying his brother's wife (Chibi, 1994). Henry, desperate for a male heir and convinced by his interpretation of the biblical text, sought to annul his marriage to Catherine only to have this request denied by the Pope Clement (Jackson & Baker, 2021). The resulting conflict between the two influential figures set the stage for the Church of England's eventual separation from the Catholic Church, effectively ending England's adherence to the papal authority (Jackson & Baker, 2021). In other words, if Catherine's miscarriages were indeed the result of Rh disease, then these cases of Rh disease may have indirectly provoked one of the most significant events in English and Catholic history.

In contrast, a prevailing theory among historians attributed Henry's infertility issues to a chronic case of syphilis, which was endemic in much of Europe at the time (Taylor, 1971). If left untreated, syphilis is known to cause infertility in both men and women by damaging the tissues of reproductive organs (Taylor, 1971). These assertions have since been challenged by the possibility that these reproduction issues may instead be attributed to a Rh blood incompatibility between Henry, who may have had Rh positive blood, and Catherine, who may have had Rh negative blood (Whitley & Kramer, 2010). Some medical historians have suggested that Rh blood incompatibility could also explain the infertility issues between Henry and his second wife, Anne Boleyn, with whom three of their four children died in utero (Whitley & Kramer, 2010). Similarly to Catherine, some medical historians contend that Henry possessed Rh positive blood whereas Anne Boleyn possessed Rh negative blood. As an aside, the sole surviving child of Anne Boleyn, Elizabeth I, eventually succeeded Mary Tudor as Queen of England.

Setting aside the complications of the English monarchy, it should be acknowledged that many medical historians recognize another early record of Rh disease, one which occurred nearly a century later in nearby France. In 1609, Louise Bourgeois, a midwife who worked in the Royal Court of the coincidentally-named Henry IV, reported on the birth and early death of a pair of twins (Liumbruno et al., 2010). In a statement to the popular press, Louise explained that the first twin had been born with hydrops, pale and bloated with fluid, and died almost immediately after birth (Bowman, 2006). The term hydrops refers to severe swelling in an unborn or newborn baby, typically caused by the accumulation of fluid (Liumbruno et al., 2010). The second twin, despite initially appearing healthier, soon became jaundiced, rigid, and developed neurological complications before dying just four days after birth (Bowman, 2006). Despite being regarded as separate conditions at the time, these symptoms are now collectively recognized as being tell-tale signs of Rh disease (Whittle, 1992).

Looking elsewhere in Europe, Drs. Erling Häggström Lundevaller and Sören Edvinsson have used the Skellefteå region of Northern Sweden as a case study to assess the potential impact of Rh disease on the perinatal death rates historically recorded in the area between the years 1860 and 1900 (2012). In their report, they noted that stillbirths and perinatal mortality were unevenly distributed across families, with a small proportion of families contributing to a large proportion of all such deaths in the region (Lundevaller & Edvinsson, 2012). In other words, it was found that there was a concentrated frequency of stillbirths in families that have previously experienced stillbirths. When compared with the distribution of the Rh negative blood type in the Skellefteå region, the clustering of stillbirths seemingly indicate that Rh disease had a considerable impact on the mortality rates observed in the region (Lundevaller & Edvinsson, 2012). While the exact causes are impossible to ascertain due to its retrospective nature, the study findings may challenge historical records of perinatal deaths, especially those which have previously been attributed to factors such as poor nutrition and insufficient sanitary measures.

Many of the historical records of Rh disease, including all those discussed so far in the chapter, seem to originate from Europe. While the apparent abundance of historical European accounts of Rh disease may be in part explained by a Eurocentric bias in academic discourse, this trend may also be accounted for by the distribution of Rh negative blood types around the world. For instance, past population studies have determined that approximately 15% of European women possess Rh negative blood, whereas Rh negative blood is only present in about 0.5% of women in East Asian populations (Visser et al., 2019). For comparison, the prevalence of Rh negative blood in Sub-Saharan African populations generally tends to be less than 5%, with one notable outlier: the population of Ethiopia (Osaro & Charles, 2010).

Recent studies have suggested that the prevalence of Rh negative blood types may be as high as 19.37% in Ethiopia, much higher than what has been previously reported in other regions of Sub-Saharan Africa (Golassa et al., 2017). This prevalence seems to be higher, around 21.31%, in the traditionally Christian populations of the Ethiopian Highlands (Golassa et al., 2017). This points us in the direction of another potential record of historical cases of Rh disease, preserved in the ethnocultural practices and traditions of certain Ethiopian Highlander populations, namely the indigenous Oromo and Amharic communities.

In Amharic communities, which form the second largest ethnic community in Ethiopia, women who have repeatedly lost newborns, either through stillbirth or neonatal death, are said to be cursed with shotelaye (Sisay et al., 2014). In these contexts, the term refers to a malicious ancestral spirit which possesses the bodies of pregnant women to kill their newborns (Sisay et al., 2014). These women often face significant discrimination, which tends to manifest in the forms of divorce, communal violence, and forced eviction from rental properties (Sisay et al., 2014). In some cases, these women are even described as *woldobela*, an Amharic term referring to 'a woman who kills children with her evil eye'.

Further evidence of the historical prevalence of Rh disease can be found in the ethnobotanical records of the Ethiopian Orthodox Church, an institution indigenous to the Ethiopian Highlands (Teklehaymanot, 2007). Ethnobotany, from which the term ethnobotanical is derived, refers to the study of the practical use of plants by local cultures and traditions (Balick & Cox, 1996). One study reviewed the medical records and manuscripts of the Debre Libanos monastery, a site of religious pilgrimage which had been established some time in the 13th century (Teklehaymanot, 2007). Speaking with several priests and nuns at the monastery, the study authors determined that there was not only a historical record of women afflicted with *shotelaye*, which are now recognized as a form of hydrops caused by Rh blood incompatibility, but there was also a record of plants which were recommended to be prescribed in its treatment (Teklehaymanot, 2007). For healing purposes, the monastery recommended the use of a shrub locally known as chifrig, *Sida schimperiana*, which was to be tied around the waist or forehead of the affected woman (Teklehaymanot, 2007).

With regards to the geographic distribution of Rh negative blood types, it's worth acknowledging that some of the highest concentrations can be found among the Basque people of the Western Pyrenees, a region straddling the Bay of Biscay along the border between Spain and France (Flores-Bello et al., 2018). Based on the data collected from the ethnic Basque communities of Spain, France, and Argentina, the prevalence of the Rh negative blood type in this population may range between 20% to nearly 50% (Touinssi et al., 2004). Prior to the development of the modern health interventions now used to prevent Rh disease, the elevated levels of Rh blood incompatibility in Basque communities may have contributed to their increased vulnerability to miscarriages and stillbirths, in turn resulting in their historically slow population growth relative to the growth seen among neighbouring ethnic communities (Touinssi et al., 2004).

Oftentimes, the high frequency of miscarriages among the Basque community may have also made them the target for accusations of witchcraft, especially in times of religious upheaval (Smith, 2000). For instance, during the 17th century Basque witch trials instigated by the Spanish Inquisition, juries frequently cited reproductive issues such as stillbirths, miscarriages, and neonatal death as evidence of witchcraft and satanism (Barstow, 1988). In these trials, an estimated 80% of the accused and 85% of the executed were women (Barstow, 1988). There have also been cases of non-Basque women blaming their own stillbirths on the actions of *mala cristianas brujas*, a term referring to witches (Rojas, 2016).

Supernatural explanations for perinatal deaths, specifically those which can be attributed to Rh disease, have historically been pervasive in different world cultures and societies. For instance, stories of the *Jinn*, a term referring to supernatural beings in Arabic and Islamic mythology, have been cited as the cause for infertility, miscarriages, and early infant deaths (Rothenberg, 2011). Some of these supernatural explanations have even survived into the modern day, as revealed in a study conducted on the causal explanations for miscarriages in Qatar (Kilshaw et al., 2017). Similarly, in the Hebrew Testament of Solomon, the demon Abyzou was said to be the cause of stillbirths and miscarriages, allegedly driven by envy as she herself was infertile (Kimball, 2019). While Abyzou is rarely recognized today, her depiction in the Hebrew Testament of Solomon is considered to be the inspiration for other beings with similar themes of infertility and stillbirth that have survived into present-day folklore and religions, most famously the demonic figure of Lilith in Jewish folklore (Kimball, 2019). Lilith continues to be a prominent figure in occultism, horror, and literature, where she continues to be associated with the occurrence of still-births and cot deaths (Kimball, 2019).

In conclusion, while modern academic circles have largely demystified its underlying biological mechanisms, there is strong evidence to suggest that Rh disease has been recognized in some capacity long before its formal identification in the late 1930s (Levine & Stetson, 1939). Historic accounts of Rh disease have existed as early as 400 BC, and there is reason to believe that the disease itself has been immortalized in the myths and traditions of various societies from Iberia to the Horn of Africa (Teklehaymanot, 2007). While the demystification of Rh disease stands as an incredible achievement, shedding light on a phenomenon that had once been feared as the work of demons and witchcraft, misinformation continues to persist in much of the world. Some of the contemporary superstitions and misconceptions surrounding Rh disease will be discussed in greater detail in "Chapter 10: How is RH Disease talked about in Society?".

This chapter primarily addresses the history of Rh disease before its formal conceptualization in academic circles. For more insight into the early breakthroughs leading up to our contemporary understanding of Rh disease, a process which only began in the last century, please refer to the next section, "Chapter 2: Who Discovered RH Disease and How Did They Do It?".

CHAPTER 2

Who Discovered RH Disease and How Did They Do It?

Written By **Rodala Aranya**

INTRODUCTION

The discovery of Rh disease took place through some key milestones over a few years. These turning points eventually concluded to create a comprehensive understanding of Rh disease. No one individual discovered the disease, but rather it was the contribution of multiple doctors resulting in a thorough understanding of the disease. To provide a clear picture of the discovery of Rh disease and all its features, we will explore five historic papers.

First, we will look at the paper of Dr. Darrow (1938), in which she is able to characterize the nature of how the disease forms. Second, an exploration will be done of a particular case published by Dr. Levine and Dr. Stetson (1939). A mother who received blood from her husband faced transfusion complications after childbirth of a stillborn fetus. Third, a brief highlight of Landsteiner and Wiener's paper will present the Rh blood group antigen (1940). Following, we will refer to Wiener and Peter (1940) and their work to explore the Rh incompatibility in blood transfusions in detail. Lastly, Levine et al.'s paper will tie in all the previous work to conclude the distinctive features of Rh disease (1941). The following sections will explore these publications in order.

1938—DR. DARROW: "ICTERUS GRAVIS (ERYTHROBLASTOSIS) NEONATORUM"

The first paper we will look at does not make any connections to Rhesus blood groups or Rh disease. Still, it does provide an excellent clinical description of Icterus Gravis Neonatorum (or erythroblastosis), which we now identify as hemolytic disease of the newborn (HDN). This is caused when the red blood cells of a newborn break down at a rapid rate, leading to the infant suffering major health complications (Baskett, 2019). The breakthrough in understanding how HDN functions came in 1938 when Dr. Darrow proposed that the baby's red cells were destroyed by an immune reaction on the mother's part.

Dr. Ruth Darrow had a personal stake in the research she was doing. In 1935, she gave birth to a son who died shortly after, suffering from erythroblastosis. Following her harrowing personal experiences, Dr. Darrow went on to research HDN extensively. In 1938, while working at the Children's Hospital in Chicago, Dr. Darrow published a detailed analysis titled, "Icterus Gravis (Erythroblastosis) Neonatorum." Her paper presented an in-depth analysis of literature, case descriptions by clinicians, and observations conducted by medical scientists (Darrow, 1938).

She theorized that frequent familial occurrence of this disease was unquestionable and concluded that the mother was always the constant factor in all cases of HDN. She also noted that in many cases, women who gave birth to infants with HDN had given birth previously, some-times to multiple infants without complications. Levine et al. (1941) touch upon this occurrence in their paper. She concluded that some sort of immune reaction had to be what was destroying the red blood cells. The fetal hemoglobin must have been immunologically different from adult hemoglobin. Through access to the maternal circulation, the mother would become actively immunized against these blood cells. The mother's body would then produce antibodies to protect itself against the foreign fetal red blood cells. While this didn't necessarily harm the mother, when the antibodies would pass through the placenta to the fetus, they would destroy the fetus's red blood cells (Darrow, 1938).

She, however, was not able to form the connection that the antigen that was causing the disease was a blood group antigen; she wrote that a difference in blood groups of the mother and child was not a factor (Baskett, 2019). Nonetheless, through her published clinical observations, Dr. Darrow arrived at an almost complete description of the nature of the disease, stating, "Antigen-antibody reaction seems to explain best all aspects of these related disorders" (Darrow, 1938, pg 37).

1939–LEVINE & STETSON: "AN UNUSUAL CASE OF INTRAGROUP AGGLUTINATION"

Following this, we see the documentation of a case later linked to erythroblastosis fetalis and Rh incompatibility by Dr. Philip Levin with Rufus E. Stetson. In 1939, they published their historic paper, titled "An unusual case of intragroup agglutination," in which they explored a rare property that was found in the blood of the mother of a stillborn fetus. As this is one of the most famous cases in the field of Rh disease, we will explore what happened in detail.

On July 12, 1937, a 25-year-old pregnant woman was admitted to Bellevue Hospital almost three months before her due date. She presented with pretibial myxedema, which is characterized by lumpiness and swelling of the lower legs. She also had a 130/90 mm Hg blood pressure, whereas a regular blood reading would be closer to 120/80 mm Hg. Her blood pressure rose to 154/106 mm Hg in about two weeks, but her symptoms slowly faded as she took bed rest. While fetal heart sounds could not be heard, there were no signs of fetal death on her X-rays. The following paragraph may be upsetting for some readers, mentioning fetal death (Levine & Stetson, 1939).

Fast forward to September 8, when she experienced labour pains and vaginal bleeding during her thirty-third week of pregnancy and was admitted to the hospital that night. She bled a significant amount before her amniotic sac ruptured (also known as one's water breaking). The delivery of a macerated fetus that showed skin and soft tissue changes—suggesting that death of the fetus transpired before delivery, possibly months earlier- was performed (Levine & Stetson, 1939)

The bleeding was finally controlled after the placenta was expelled from the birth canal. She was given her first blood transfusion of 500 c.c. from her husband. They were both blood group O. Within ten minutes, she felt an ache in her legs and head, and after twelve hours, a piece of her placenta passed, and she began bleeding heavily once more. Later, another blood transfusion of 750 c.c. was given without any severe reactions. Unfortunately, she started bleeding once again, and a hysterectomy was performed, during which she received her third blood transfusion. Almost twenty hours after her first blood transfusion, she had lost 8 ounces of blood and discharged bloody urine (Levine & Stetson, 1939).

As they performed tests, they found a rare property in the patient's blood that would lead to the discovery of Rh disease. Her reports showed an iso-agglutination of moderate activity. Essentially, this meant that she had produced antibodies that caused agglutination (the development of antigen complexes in the form of particle clumps) of the red blood cells. Even though the patient and her husband were both in the blood group O, tests showed that over 80 percent of her blood had been agglutinated. That night, she had suffered from a very severe hemolytic reaction from the blood transfusion. The reaction occurs when the person's immune system destroys red blood cells given during the transfusion. In this case, her husband's cells have been attacked by her immune system (Levine & Stetson, 1939).

With the careful assistance of the Blood Transfusion Betterment Association, she went on to receive six more blood transfusions from donors who were meticulously selected. With no reactions whatsoever, she eventually saw a full recovery. The remaining part of the report explores the findings of the serum, which is the fluid component of blood that includes all proteins. It is important to note that while later works would link the death of the fetus and the mother's blood incompatibility, Levine and Stetson's conclusions only concerned that of the patient's blood and the transfusion reaction (Levine & Stetson, 1939).

The test results highlighted that only 8/50 group O donors were compatible and did not react with the patient's blood serum. In another test, only 13/54 group O donors did not react with the patient's blood serum. In total, only 21/104 group O donors were compatible, and her serum agglutinated with around 80 percent of the blood specimens. Levine and Stetson both proposed that perhaps this was an unexpected blood incompatibility. Two months later, they found that the serum still displayed agglutination but at a milder level (Levine & Stetson, 1939).

They reported that the agglutination became present several weeks after repeated blood transfusions. However, they did acknowledge that in their patient's case, the iso-agglutination had to have been present when she was given the first transfusion from her husband. Taking into consideration that their patient was carrying a fetus that had passed away several months ago in utero, they concluded that the disintegrating cells of the fetus must have been responsible for both the symptoms that the patient experienced—such as high fever and bloody urine—and the iso-immunization she presented. In previous tests, the immunizing property was not displayed in the patient's blood, so Levine and Stetson theorized that this dominant property must have been in the blood or tissue of the fetus, inherited from the father. It must have been responsible for the production of the antibodies (Levine & Stetson, 1939). Here, they stopped short in identifying what the property was. In the following paper, Landsteiner and Wiener (1940) do just that.

1940—LANDSTEINER & WIENER: "AN AGGLUTINABLE FACTOR IN HUMAN BLOOD RECOGNIZED BY IMMUNE SERA FOR RHESUS BLOOD"

In 1940, Karl Landsteiner and Alexander S. Wiener made a connection to an earlier discovery they had made. Before we explore the findings of their 1940 paper, let's briefly summarize their previous results. In this study, they had been raising immune sera in animals. Immune sera refer to a serum that contains antibodies, which the animals were making due to the injection of red blood cells in their tissues from other species. They were successfully able to show that rabbits who had been injected with the blood of Rhesus monkeys had formed antibodies that agglutinated cells that carried the human M antigen, which is also present in the monkeys (Levine, 1984).

As discussed in the previous sections, Darrow (1938) explored a potential cause of the disease, while Levine and Stetson (1939) found a new type of blood incompatibility between the mother and fetus, resulting in antibodies. These studies had come just short of naming it. In their 1940 publication, Landsteiner and Wiener published the article introducing the human blood group antigen, Rh. The report explained that serum that contained Rh would agglutinate with the majority of other human blood. Thus, another human blood group antigen was discovered (Landsteiner & Wiener, 1940).

1940—WIENER & PETERS: "HEMOLYTIC REACTIONS FOLLOWING TRANSFUSIONS OF BLOOD OF THE HOMOLOGOUS GROUP, WITH THREE CASES IN WHICH THE SAME AGGLUTINOGEN WAS RESPONSIBLE"

The next paper written by Dr. Wiener and Dr. Peters is of great value to understanding Rh disease. The article published in 1940 is titled, "Hemolytic reactions following transfusions of the blood of the homologous group, with three cases in which the same agglutinogen was responsible." They detail three reactions that occurred after transfusions of donor-recipients who had the same ABO type. This is a type of blood group classification (Wiener & Peters, 1940).

Wiener and Peters start their paper by acknowledging that certain patients would have transfusion reactions from time to time despite belonging to the same ABO group. Their studies show "intra-group" reactions where the antibodies in the patients reacted with the donor cells, which they concluded were a reaction against the Rh factor. The details of the three cases are described below, with emphasis on the first case as it led to their most crucial breakthrough (Wiener & Peters, 1940).

In the first case, they observe a 52-year-old woman who was admitted to the surgical service of Mercy Hospital on August 13, 1939, with a solitary ruptured ulcer. The day after her operation, the patient was given their first blood transfusion at 500 c.c. of group O blood and their second one at 300 c.c. Over the next few days, she received three more transfusions in the span of eight days, all from different group O donors, who had been cross-matched to be from the same blood group (Wiener & Peters, 1940).

She showed no visceral reactions, but following the week after the operation, the patient had a continuous high temperature of 103 degrees F. During her last transfusion, her fever rose to 104 degrees F. The next day she exhibited various deteriorating conditions. She suffered from hemoglobinuria, which is the abnormal presence of hemoglobin in urine and had very little urine output in general. She also became notably jaundiced—where the skin, whites of her eyes and mucous membranes turned yellow. Her hemoglobin count fell drastically, reaching as low as 46 percent. The patient passed away four days after the onset of her last transfusion reaction (Wiener & Peters, 1940).

Wiener received the blood from the patient after her last transfusion and, following her death, ran some tests. This confirmed that both the patient and donor had belonged to group O. Still, it also showed that clumping occurred when the patient's serum was added to the donor's cell and refrigerated for two hours. This confirmed that the patient's serum must contain special agglutinations, different from known isoagglutination, and the blood was incompatible (Wiener & Peters, 1940).

They then tested blood samples from many different group O individuals with the patient's serum. It was discovered that the majority of blood was agglutinated by the antibody, unrelated to any previously known agglutinogens. Remarkably, they noted, "'the reactions coincided with those given by certain anti-Rhesus immune rabbit sera recently described by Landsteiner and Wiener which define an agglutinable property of human blood designated as Rh" (Wiener & Peters, 1940, pg 2309). This was a historic correlation as it was the first publication to tie together transfusion incompatibility with the Rh factor (Levine, 1984).

They presumed that the patient must have been Rh-negative, and the blood given was Rh-positive. The repeated transfusions had created the production of Rh antibodies, responsible for her death. They concluded, "the' agglutinable property demonstrated with the patient's serum is identical with Rh" (Wiener & Peters, 1940, pg 2310). The principles underlying the reactions of the three patients were easy to understand following this understanding.

The second case follows a patient who had received four transfusions from two donors, all group A, and suffered complications similar to the first case. This patient did improve by the end of their stay. It was found in testing that the patient was Rh-negative, and the blood for the first and last transfusion was incompatible as it was Rh-positive. The second and third transfusions were from an Rh-negative donor, so their blood was compatible. The first transfusion had sensitized the patent, while the following two had no effect. The fourth transfusion had been what caused antibodies to be created in the patient's blood. They concluded the reactions were identical and contained the antibody produced by the Rh factor (Wiener & Peters, 1940).

They followed this case by testing the serum of patient 1 and patient 2 with 11 individuals. Their findings showed that only 14 people's blood did not cause the blood to agglutinate in the anti-Rh sera. They write,

"Our findings presented above confirm the occurrence of hemolytic reactions after transfusions of the blood of the proper group, due to agglutinogens unrelated to the four blood groups" (Wiener & Peters, 1940, pg 2317).

The third case, which took place in 1935, shows that not all unexplained transfusion reactions could be traced to the formation of Rh-positive antibodies in an Rh-negative individual. The details of this case are beyond the scope of this book (Wiener & Peters, 1940).

Wiener and Peters made another interesting observation. Building off information accumulated in previous years, they noted that hemolytic reactions that occurred in patients who had never received a blood transfusion were women who had recently given birth or suffered a miscarriage (Wiener & Peters, 1940). They refer to the Levine and Stetson (1939) paper where the patient, after a stillbirth, had received blood transfusions from her husband and experienced a hemolytic reaction. They suggest that an Rh-negative mother carrying an Rh-positive fetus may react by producing antibodies if the placenta cannot provide a sufficient barrier between the two (Wiener & Peters, 1940).

This paper was truly ground-breaking in that it brought together the observations of animal and human testing to establish Rh incompatibility while also foreshadowing future conclusions. However, the article mainly focused on the Rh incompatibility transfusion reactions rather than on Rh hemolytic disease of the newborn. (Stockman, 2001). This will be all tied together when we explore the following paper.

1941–LEVINE ET AL.: "THE ROLE OF ISOIMMUNIZATION IN THE PATHOGENESIS OF ERYTHROBLASTOSIS FETALIS"

In the following year, Levine, alongside a few scientists put the entire pathophysiological puzzle together. In this paper, they were able to bring together the previous knowledge of Rh groups, blood incompatibility, and transfusion reactions and combine it with the understanding of the hemolytic disease of the newborn, establishing a definitive description of the nature of Rh disease. The researchers established the reaction that could occur between Rh-negative mothers pregnant with a fetus carrying Rh-positive red blood cells (Levine et al., 1941). Drawing from many different observations, the paper provides an exceptionally comprehensive analysis of the nature of Rh disease.

The first point of exploration was that of the patient from Levine and Stetson's paper (1939). Three years after her agglutination reaction from the transfusions she had received, the patient's blood and her husband were tested. It was discovered that she was Rh-negative while her husband had been Rh-positive. They theorized that a pregnant woman who is Rh-negative and has a child with an Rh-positive man could create anti-Rh agglutination due to immunization by the Rh fetal red blood cells. The subsequent passage of maternal agglutination and antibodies through the placenta resulted in erythroblastosis fetalis (Levine et al., 1941).

The central part of the paper was the examination of 153 mothers who had given birth to children with HDN. It showed that 90 percent of the women were Rh-negative, a much more significant percentage than the average of 15 percent in the general U.S. population. It was also found that the husbands and infants were always Rh-positive (Levine et al., 1941).

Levine et al. also furthered two reasons that only one of several pregnancies would result in an infant with HDN. The first reason could be that the father may be heterozygous for the gene. There are different versions of genes, and each is called an allele. A person inherits two alleles for every gene, one from their father and one from their mother. If a person (in this case, the infant's father with HDN) has two different versions, they have a heterozygous genotype for that gene. This means that there is around a 50 percent chance that his offspring will be Rh-positive. Another reason they presented was that more than one pregnancy with an Rh-positive fetus might be necessary for the mother to create a sufficient amount of isoimmunization (Levin et al.al, 1941).

To conclude their paper, Levine et al. provided a few key takeaways of what we now recognize to be all the features of Rh disease. In the cases that they examined, 93 percent showed that erythroblastosis fetalis resulted from iso-immunization of an Rh-negative mother by the Rh factor in the fetus' red blood cells. The antibodies created by the mother attack the susceptible red blood cells of the fetus and causes hemolysis of its blood. In the remaining 7 percent of cases, it was found that blood factors not related to Rh were responsible for isoimmunization. They also advised that women with high incidences of recurrent miscarriages and stillbirths and who later had reactions from transfusion may have been sensitized to the Rh factor, and their blood type should be investigated. They further asserted that transfusion reactions always tended to be associated with pregnancies and could be prevented using a modified cross-matching test and Rh-negative donors. Lastly, they recommended that testing for agglutination for the Rh factor would be instrumental in the diagnosis of erythroblastosis fetalis (Levine et al., 1941).

A NOTE ON THE RHESUS FACTOR AND RH GROUPING

For accuracy, it should be acknowledged that it was later discovered that the Rhesus antibody first described by Landsteiner and Wiener in the 1940s concerning animal serum is not identical to the antigens produced by humans. By that point, most literature had been using terms such as "Rhesus group," and it felt impractical to change the name of the human antibody. To this day, we retain the term Rhesus factor and refer to the group as the "Rh blood group system" and the antibody as "anti-Rh" (Stockman, 2001).

CONCLUSION

It is evident that the discovery of Rh disease was the work of multiple researchers, all of whom acknowledged and built off each other's research to produce papers that would eventually lead to a conclusive understanding of the disease. We can see the puzzle pieces come together and create a picture detailing the story of Rh disease.

Dr. Darrow (1937) was the first to suggest that the cause of HDN may be due to an iso-immunization in the mother that attacked the fetus's red blood cells. Levine and Stetson (1939) published the account of a mother who had reacted to blood transfusions from her husband following a stillbirth, showing agglutination of the red blood cells. Landsteiner and Wiener (1940) were the first to name this human antigen the Rh factor. Wiener then partnered with Peters (1940) to detail accounts of transfusion reactions of agglutination due to blood incompatibility based on the Rh factor. Lastly, Levine et al. (1941) were able to tie all the previous conclusions concerning HDN to propose all the features of what we now know as Rh disease.

Following these historic developments, the medical community saw further expansion in terms of diagnosis and treatments, which were applauded as outstanding advances in medicine. These understandings culminated two decades later. In the following chapter, we explore how these findings contributed to the greater knowledge of hemolytic diseases and, in doing so, allowed for more accurate diagnosis and treatment.

CHAPTER 3

How Did the Discovery of RH Disease Impact the Study of Hemolytic Diseases?

*Written By **Pareesa Ali***

INTRODUCTION

As discussed in the previous two chapters, the discovery of Rhesus disease was a major finding, especially in the field of hemolytic diseases. Understanding Rhesus disease and the subsequent study into its treatments contributed to an overall understanding regarding hemolytic diseases. This chapter sets out to discuss the significance of Rhesus disease and the ways in which its discovery impacted the field of hemolytic diseases as a whole.

To begin, let's start with the importance of understanding blood types. Next, we'll move on to discussing hemolytic diseases, which will then lead us to understanding a specific hemolytic disease known as Rhesus disease. Following this, we'll cover our understanding of Rhesus disease with regards to the complications it is associated with. Finally, we'll finish by going over how significant the discovery of Rhesus disease has been in the overall field of hemolytic diseases. Now, as a refresher, all individuals are born with a specific blood type; either type A, B, AB or O (Stanford Children's Health). Each individual also has a protein on the outside of their red blood cells, known as the Rhesus factor, or Rh factor, which can be classified as either positive or negative (Sarwar & Sridhar,

2020). The Rh factor is genetically inherited, which means you inherit it from your parents. Inheriting the protein means you are Rh positive, while not having inherited the protein means you are Rh negative. The Rh factor is found in the blood of 85% of White individuals and 95% of Black individuals (Oyelowo, 2007). Moreover, your blood type can act as a risk factor and it can be used to predict your predisposition to certain diseases or health effects (Miao et al., 2014). For example, a meta-analysis conducted in 2014 revealed that Caucasians with blood type A had a higher risk of breast cancer than other Caucasians (Miao et al., 2014). The reason behind this variance is due to the presence of blood group antigens (Miao et al., 2014). An antigen can be thought of as a substance on the surface of your cells that triggers your immune system into producing antibodies (Groot et al., 2020). For instance, with regards to your blood type, blood type A has A antigens, while blood type AB has both A and B antigens (Groot et al., 2020). Blood group antigens can influence the inflammatory response seen in the body, as certain antigens are associated with higher levels of inflammation (Miao et al., 2014). Furthermore, an individual inherits their blood type and Rh factor from their parents. However, an incompatibility in blood types or Rh factors between a pregnant mother and her child can have severe consequences for the developing fetus.

HEMOLYTIC DISEASES

Hemolytic diseases are blood disorders defined by the destruction of red blood cells at a rate that is faster than the rate of production of these cells (Dean & Dean, 2005). Certain hemolytic diseases are associated with blood types and blood factors, specifically the Rh factor. While the presence of the Rh factor has no negative consequences for an individual, an incompatibility in blood types between a pregnant mother and her baby can have dire consequences for the developing fetus. For instance, if an Rh negative mother is pregnant with an Rh positive fetus, due to the fetus having an Rh positive father, then this can have severe consequences for the fetus. A detrimental consequence of this incompatibility is a hemolytic disease known as the hemolytic disease of the newborn (HDN), which was previously a significant contributor of fetal loss and deaths among newborn babies (Dean & Dean, 2005).

This disease is the result of the newborn's red blood cells being attacked by antibodies from the mother (Dean & Dean, 2005). These antibodies responsible for destroying the fetal red blood cells can either occur naturally in the mother's body, or can develop after an event such as blood transfusions or pregnancy (Basu et al., 2011). The disease is represented by four disorders: hydrops, or severe swelling, jaundice, anemia, and erythroblastosis, a severe type of anemia (Baskett, 2019). The breakdown of fetal red blood cells by maternal antibodies leads to prolonged jaundice and anemia, causing newborns to be sick and unstable at birth (Roberts, 2008).

In addition, prior to the development of any preventative measures, affected fetuses had a mortality rate of up to 50% (Ree et al., 2017). Thus, the discovery of this disease shed light on the importance of matching blood types for transfusions, and testing blood type compatibility between a pregnant mother and her child. The treatment for this disease will be discussed further in chapter 9. Overall, understanding blood type compatibility and any potential risk of hemolytic disease of the newborn is important for all individuals, especially those who are, or are trying to get pregnant.

UNDERSTANDING RHESUS DISEASE

In particular, a specific type of HDN is triggered by the mother and fetus having different Rh blood groups, causing a disease known as Rhesus disease (Dean & Dean, 2005). Prior to the discovery of the Rhesus protein, HDN was a significant cause of perinatal mortality (Basu et al., 2011). Rhesus disease, or Rh disease, is a hemolytic disease, which is named after the process of hemolysis (Dean & Dean, 2005). Hemolysis involves the breaking down and destruction of red blood cells (Dean & Dean, 2005). The most common cause of Rhesus disease is when an Rh negative mother has a baby with an Rh positive father, leading to an incompatibility in blood types between the mother and fetus (Sarwar & Sridhar, 2020). Another potential cause of Rhesus disease is through the transfusion of Rh positive blood into an Rh negative mother (Traut & McIvor, 1946).

This can be problematic if the baby's Rh positive red blood cells mix with the Rh negative mother's red blood cells during pregnancy (Sarwar & Sridhar, 2020). This is because an individual's immune system produces antibodies when they sense a foreign substance in the body. Therefore, the mother's immune system will view the baby's Rh positive red blood cells as a foreign object, and will respond by making antibodies to destroy these cells (Sarwar & Sridhar, 2020). In Rh disease, maternal antibodies attack and destroy the baby's red blood cells in the womb through the process of hemolysis (Hemolytic Disease of the Newborn). The specific process occurs when the Rh positive blood in the fetus, inherited from the father, makes its way into the mother's circulation during pregnancy or delivery (Oyelowo, 2007). The mother's immune system, being Rh negative, makes Rh positive antibodies (Oyelowo, 2007). This is harmful because the antibodies will launch an attack against the fetus, destroying the fetal red blood cells (Oyelowo, 2007).

This destruction of red blood cells can lead to anemia, which can have harmful consequences including fatal brain damage, due to the lack of critical oxygen that the fetus has access to (Oyelowo, 2007). This attack causes an incompatibility between the mother's and baby's blood while the baby is still in the womb (Dean & Dean, 2005). As the antibodies destroy the cells, the baby gets sick, causing a disease known as erythroblastosis fetalis during pregnancy (Sarwar & Sridhar, 2020). After the baby's birth, the disease is called HDN (Hemolytic Disease of the Newborn).

COMPLICATIONS OF RHESUS DISEASE

The presence of the Rhesus factor has no complications for an Rh positive individual; however, Rhesus disease triggered in Rh negative pregnant mothers can have major complications for their unborn babies (Hemolytic Disease of the Newborn). These complications include fetal heart failure, fluid retention and swelling, and stillbirth (Hemolytic Disease of the Newborn). Hemolysis of the fetal red blood cells can cause major complications such as severe fetal anemia and hyperbilirubinemia, which can lead to neurological damage or death (Sarwar & Sridhar, 2020). More than half of fetuses or newborns with Rh disease die; while those who survive suffer from severe disease and significant brain damage (Pegoraro et al., 2020). As previously mentioned, a severe hemolytic disease triggered by Rh disease is known as erythroblastosis fetalis, and is characterized by jaundice and severe hemolytic anemia (Sarwar & Sridhar, 2020).

Moreover, severe hemolytic anemia in the fetus is defined by the baby's red blood cells being destroyed faster than they can be replaced (Sarwar & Sridhar, 2020). The effects of this can lead to severe jaundice, liver failure and even heart failure (Sarwar & Sridhar, 2020). The intermediate effects of these conditions are characterized in infants as lethargy, irritability, fever, high-pitched cry, and a lack of feeding (Smits-Wintjens et al., 2008). The advanced stages of disease are demonstrated by a shrill cry, no feeding, coma, and even seizures and death (Smits-Wintjens et al., 2008). Lastly, the chronic stage involves infants developing cerebral palsy, hearing problems, and psychomotor handicaps, which the child will suffer from for the rest of their life (Smits-Wintjens et al., 2008). While all of these effects are incredibly damaging for the infant, proper and timely care and treatment can offset these effects and allow for appropriate development of the newborn (Alaqeel, 2019). Thus, understanding hemolytic diseases is an incredibly important advancement for decreasing risk of fetal and newborn deaths.

SIGNIFICANCE OF THE DISCOVERY
Luckily, Rh disease is now preventable due to the scientific advancements of modern medicine. A major part of preventing HDN involves determining the Rh status of the mother and seeking timely preventative

measures during pregnancy (Dean & Dean, 2005). 98% of HDN cases are due to Rh and ABO blood type incompatibilities between the mother and fetus, while 2% of HDN cases are due to the presence of irregular antibodies, such as those caused by blood transfusions (Weinstein, 1982). This exemplifies the need for blood banks to screen blood transfusions for pregnant women to ensure they are entirely compatible. Understanding Rh disease is the primary step towards decreasing the prevalence of hemolytic diseases.

Additionally, the screening of all pregnant patients for the presence of irregular antibodies can alert them to any potential risk of HDN (Mollison & Cutbush, 1951). It can also allow for time to ensure the laboratory can find a matching and compatible blood donor, in the event of needing an emergency blood transfusion (Mollison & Cutbush, 1951). Moreover, paternal testing for the Rh antigen is also a necessary step to help manage the health of the patient and their unborn child (Mollison & Cutbush, 1951). Therefore, timely Rh screening of the parents, along with treatment with antibodies known as Rh immunoglobulins is an extremely effective treatment for battling Rh incompatibility (Sarwar & Sridhar, 2020). A treatment for preventing HDN, which will be discussed further in chapter 9, involves removing the maternal antibodies responsible for attacking the fetal red blood cells (Dean & Dean, 2005). This treatment can essentially reverse the risk of HDN and improve the chances of a successful and healthy pregnancy and delivery. The transfusion of these antibodies can lead to a 92% survival rate for the fetus (Harman et al., 1983). Studying this disease provides an opportunity for understanding the field of hemolytic diseases, as other hemolytic diseases follow a similar pathogenesis of destroying red blood cells through the process of hemolysis.

SIGNIFICANCE IN THE FIELD OF HEMOLYTIC DISEASES

Furthermore, hemolytic diseases are generally classified by an abnormally short life span of circulating red blood cells (Motulsky et al., 1954). Other hereditary blood diseases include hereditary elliptocytosis, thalassemia major, and sickle cell anemia, diseases which are also characterized by diminishing red blood cells (Motulsky et al., 1954). The classification of these diseases with regards to familial hemolytic diseases is similar in certain ways. These diseases are also marked by a decreased life span of red blood cells; however, patients with these diseases may live normal lives. On the other hand, hemolytic diseases are marked by their genetic inheritance patterns and the destruction of red blood cells they cause. Another hemolytic disease, hemolytic anemia, is classified similarly to HDN as it causes the increased destruction of red blood cells (Noronha, 2016).

In contrast, however, hemolytic anemia can either be caused by congenital or acquired red blood cell abnormalities (Noronha, 2016). Moreover, since hemolytic diseases involve the destruction of red blood cells, this leads to a decreased concentration of hemoglobin in the fetal blood (Mollison & Cutbush, 1951). Hemoglobin is the protein found in red blood cells which is responsible for carrying oxygen throughout the body (Mollison & Cutbush, 1951). A decreased level of hemoglobin is closely associated with a decreased chance of survival for the infant (Mollison & Cutbush, 1951). Another disease similar to HDN in fetuses or newborns is known as fetal or neonatal alloimmune thrombocytopenia (Brojer et al., 2016). This disease is also caused by the presence of Rh antibodies; however, it is mainly characterized by platelet destruction, which are blood cells responsible for making your blood clot after injury (Brojer et al., 2016). Alloimmune thrombocytopenia puts the fetus or newborn at an increased risk for intracranial hemorrhage, also known as a brain bleed (Brojer et al., 2016). This can result in lifelong disability and even death (Brojer et al., 2016). Therefore, understanding HDN and Rhesus disease is necessary for reducing infant mortality rates, as there are other diseases who act in similar ways to Rhesus disease.

For instance, the preventative measures put in place for ensuring Rh factor compatibility for blood transfusions has been applied to ABO blood group incompatibilities as well(Berentsen & Tjønnfjord, 2012).

This has allowed for a reduction in the prevalence of ABO-related hemolytic diseases in newborns (Berentsen & Tjønnfjord, 2012). Learning about the Rh factor has helped scientists build a crucial understanding about the need for performing blood type and antibody screenings to ensure compatibility with the patient (Berentsen & Tjønnfjord, 2012). Overall, the discovery and understanding of HDN and Rhesus disease has provided a deeper understanding of how hemolytic diseases are classified and can be prevented, which has had a profound impact on the field of hemolytic diseases.

CONCLUSION

Prior to the discovery of the Rh protein and the importance of maternal and fetal Rh compatibility, HDN was a significant cause of perinatal mortality (Basu et al., 2011). Approximately four decades ago, HDN was thought to be synonymous with Rhesus disease, a common cause of infant mortality (Basu et al., 2011). Therefore, discovering the Rhesus factor and Rh incompatibility was a huge revelation in the field of hemolytic diseases. Moving on to the current world, ABO blood type incompatibility between mothers and infants is now the greatest cause of HDN (Basu et al., 2011). ABO hemolytic disease occurs most commonly now in infants of blood types A or B who are born to type O mothers (Basu et al., 2011).

The impact of this understanding of hemolytic diseases has allowed for the production of effective preventative measures for this type of HDN. These preventative measures involve testing maternal and paternal blood types prior to or during pregnancy (Baskett, 2019). Timely blood type testing, along with screening protocols during pregnancy, have allowed for the management of Rhesus disease and hemolytic diseases of the newborn (Baskett, 2019). However, despite this incredible scientific advancement, only half of pregnant women worldwide receive this preventative treatment (Pegoraro et al., 2020). In fact, a previous study found that complications from Rhesus disease were linked to the deaths of at least 50,000 fetuses and 114,000 newborns worldwide each year (Pegoraro et al., 2020). However, the global burden of Rh disease now resides primarily in lower-income countries (Pegoraro et al., 2020). This will be discussed further in chapters 8 and 11. All in all, the discovery of Rhesus disease has been a major contributor to our overall understanding of hemolytic diseases. Understanding how blood types and inherited genetic factors can influence the field of hemolytic diseases is a significant step forward for the eradication of these diseases. The mechanism of Rhesus disease has demonstrated the importance of testing blood types during pregnancy, for both the mother and the father, and the significance of screening protocols for ensuring a healthy pregnancy and delivery of the fetus. The upcoming chapters will discuss Rhesus disease in more detail, from the biological mechanisms behind it, to treatment and the overall significance of learning more about this disease.

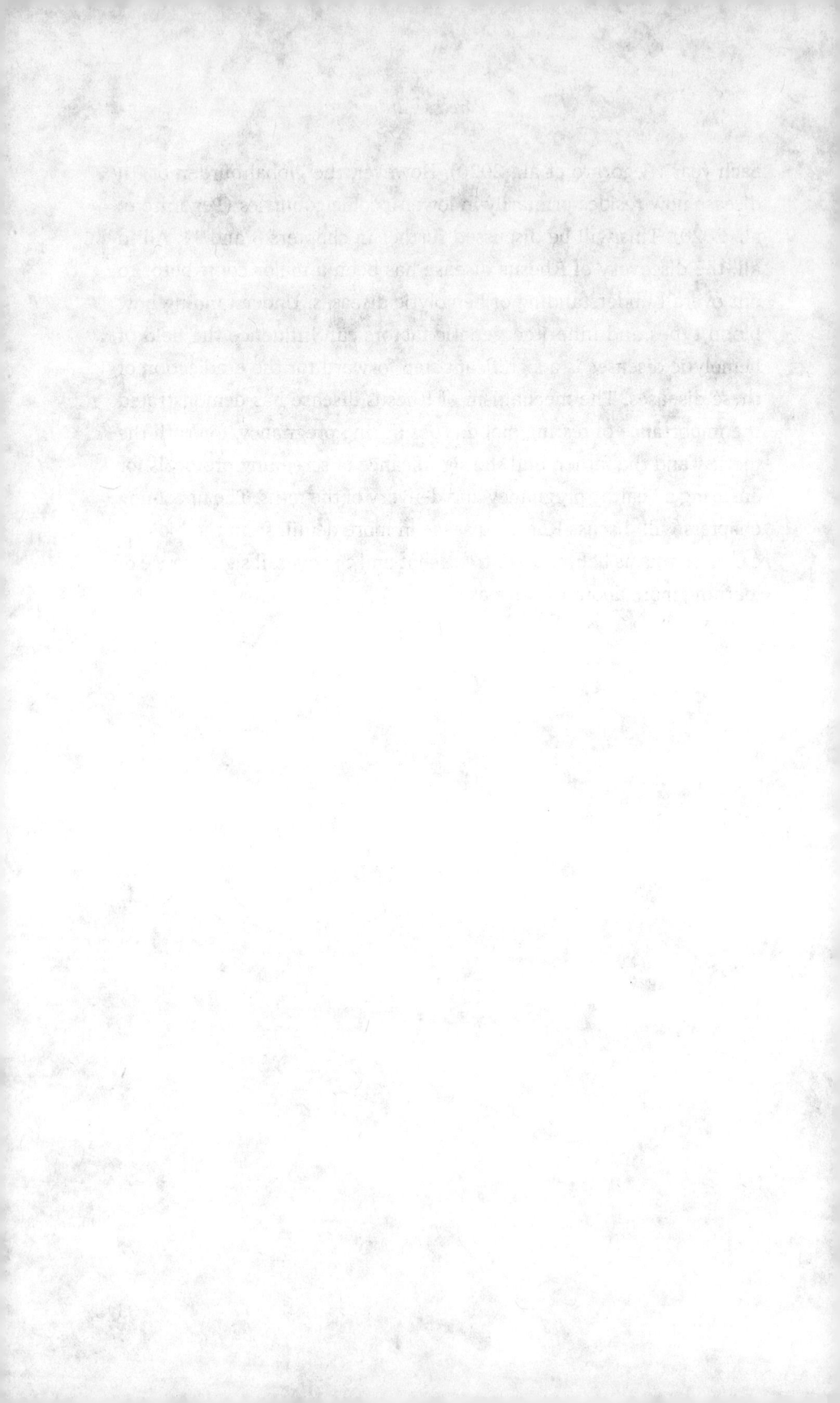

CHAPTER 4

What is RH disease?

*Written By **Dhwani Bhadresa***

THE AIM OF THIS CHAPTER is to provide background information and knowledge about Rhesus disease. This chapter begins with classifications of the disease, followed by the statistical prevalence of Rh and discusses possible causes for the condition. Additionally, evidence on symptoms and indicators of Rh are discussed. Subsequently, the importance of prevention and at-risk population are highlighted. It is important to note this chapter discusses sensitive material and topics on pregnancy and fetal death.

Rhesus disease is classified as a hemolytic disease of the newborn (HDN) (Westhoff, 2007). This is a type of blood disorder and has to do with incompatibility of blood types between the fetus and the mother (Westhoff, 2007).

The prevalence of individuals that are impacted by Rhesus disease on a global scale is approximately 276 births for every 100,000 births (Costumbrado et al., 2021). In developed countries, there is a reduced prevalence of Rh disease, with only 2.5 births for every 100,000 births. This is due to an advanced level of care in terms of the treatment of infants and newborns in these developed countries (Costumbrado et al., 2021).

In 1971, a study was conducted among Walker's community to see the prevalence of haemolytic diseases of newborns (Zipursky & Paul, 2011). Walker observed that approximately 14% of pregnancies were stillbirths (Zipursky & Paul, 2011).Among the births that survived, around 30 % were estimated to have moderate conditions which could develop into excessive levels of bilirubin in the blood known as hyperbilirubinemia (Zipursky & Paul, 2011). Brain injury, damage or death can occur if this condition is left untreated (Zipursky & Paul, 2011). In addition, another 30 % were deemed to have severe disease that could be deadly if there was no treatment provided (Zipursky & Paul, 2011). Nearly 40% did not require any form of treatment (Zipursky & Paul, 2011). From this population analysis of pregnancies, it is determined that almost 50% of newborns who are without treatment for hemolytic disease of the newborn will either pass away or have brain damage (Zipursky & Paul, 2011). The findings that were conducted in a 1971 study by Walker were similarly observed in Manitoba, Canada in regards to the prevalence of HDN within scientific studies. (Zipursky & Paul, 2011). These statistics illustrate how widespread hemolytic diseases in newborn children are.

Over the years, this disease has complicated the process of pregnancy (Westhoff, 2007). A correlation was determined between Rh disease and stimulation of an immune response. The connection was established due to observing negative consequences of both fetus and mother (Westhoff, 2007). This was concluded when a stillborn fetus was delivered. In addition researchers found negative impacts of blood transfer between father and mother (Westhoff, 2007). When understanding the effect of the immune system on Rh disease, this helps determine the potential causes for the condition.

There are two primary causes that are associated with Rh diseases. The first is the difference and exposure of blood type between a pregnant mother and fetus which can lead to serious medical side effects and complications during pregnancy (Sarwar & Citla Sridhar, 2021).The second lesser known cause of RH, which typically occurs during emergency situations, is when individuals have lost blood due to injuries requiring blood transfusion between Rh positive and Rh negative blood (Sarwar & Citla Sridhar, 2021). In situations when individuals are harmed or injured, blood transfusion is the process in which donated blood is transferred into the body under medical supervision.

When a woman is pregnant and has Rh-negative blood, and the fetus is Rh-positive, this can lead to RH disease (Sarwar & Citla Sridhar, 2021). This disease is caused when the fetus has a rhesus antigen onits red blood cells. Antigens are different proteins found on the surface of cells.

The exposure between the two different blood types, Rh-negative from the mother and Rh-positive blood cells from the fetus, can happen during a c-section or an ectopic pregnancy, as well as many other scenarios (Sarwar & Citla Sridhar, 2021).

In these circumstances, there is mixing of two different blood types (Rh positive & and Rh negative), and this leads to the mother developing anti-D antibodies, in her body (Sarwar & Sridhar, 2021). Antibodies are proteins created by an immune reaction response, triggered by antigens (Westhoff, 2007). When both the antigen and antibody are bound together, it results in an immune response to demolish foreign substances to the body (Westhoff, 2007). This leads to isoimmunization, which is the incompatibility between the maternal blood type and the fetus, and results in an immune response in the production of antibodies in the mother that harm and destroy the fetal blood cells (Sarwar & Citla Sridhar, 2021).

The Rhesus factor is associated with red blood cells and is a surface antigen which can determine if individuals are Rh negative or positive (Sarwar & Citla Sridhar, 2021). This is dependent on the D antigen, and whether this specific antigen is present or absent on red blood cells (Sarwar & Citla Sridhar, 2021). The D antigen is primarily responsible for the development of Rh disease because of its heightened capability to stimulate an immune response in the mother's body, classified as increased immunogenicity (Sarwar & Citla Sridhar, 2021).

In order to understand how individuals can be Rh positive or negative it is important to understand blood group classifications. The two that will be mentioned are the ABO and rhesus systems (Mitra et al., 2014). Every individual falls under one of these blood types: A , B, O, AB and this is labelled for the ABO system (*Rh Disease—Health Encyclopedia—University of Rochester Medical Center*, n.d.) and under the rhesus system, individuals are classified as either Rh positive or Rh negative (Mitra et al., 2014). If the Rh factor protein is present on the red blood cell this is indicative of individuals being Rh positive. The Rh negative blood type occurs when there is no protein (Rh factor) on the surface of the red blood cells. There are upwards of fifty antigens correlated with Rh blood types, the following are commonly determined: D, E, C, e, and c (Sarwar & Citla Sridhar, 2021).

Rhesus disease impacts the baby. Thus, the mother will not experience symptoms, while the baby will (*Rh Disease—Health Encyclopedia—University of Rochester Medical Center*, n.d.). It is important to recognize that symptoms associated with Rh disease will differ on a case-by-case basis depending on the baby and pregnancy (*Rh Disease—Health Encyclopedia—University of Rochester Medical Center,* n.d.). Certain factors that can influence Rh disease can be genetic blood type, previous pregnancies with a history of Rh, and paternal factors (*Rhesus Disease*, 2017).

During pregnancy, the fetus may have a larger than normal spleen, heart, and liver (*Rh Disease—Health Encyclopedia—University of Rochester Medical Center*, n.d.). In addition, there may be fluid buildup in the fetus, specifically in the lungs, stomach, and scalp (*Rh Disease —Health Encyclopedia—University of Rochester Medical Center*, n.d.). This type of extra fluid in the body is an indication of another condition, hydrops fetalis (*Rh Disease—Health Encyclopedia—University of Rochester Medical Center,* n.d.). This occurs from irregular amounts of fluid in the fetus and can cause serious amounts of swelling (*Rh Disease—Health Encyclopedia—University of Rochester Medical Center,* n.d.). Health complications that are associated with hydrops fetalis are miscarriages, and fetal death following 20 weeks of pregnancy(Vanaparthy & Mahdy, 2021).

One serious complication of Rh disease is the breakdown of fetal red blood cells which activates the release of a yellow substance known as bilirubin (*Rh Disease—Health Encyclopedia—University of Rochester Medical Center,* n.d.). This release of bilirubin is a potential cause for the colour of amniotic fluid to be yellow (*Rh Disease—Health Encyclopedia—University of Rochester Medical Center,* n.d.). While undergoing pregnancy, the amniotic fluid is a liquid that is bordering around the fetus and thus a symptom of Rh is yellowing of the amniotic fluid (*Rh Disease—Health Encyclopedia—University of Rochester Medical Center,* n.d.). Due to the increase in bilirubin, mechanisms for reduction can be exchange transfusion and phototherapy (Dean, 2005). If there is excessive levels of bilirubin in newborns this can be potentially toxic to brain cells and immediate treatment can be beneficial for protection against further damage. (*Infant Jaundice —Symptoms and Causes,* n.d.).

Another common symptom during pregnancy is that the fetus may become anemic, or deficient in iron (*Rhesus Disease—Symptoms,* 2017). Anemia develops due to the breakdown of red blood cells by the mother's antibodies (*Rhesus Disease—Symptoms,* 2017). In fetuses with anemia, the speed at which the blood travels will increase and the blood will become thinner (*Rhesus Disease—Symptoms,* 2017). In situations in which the anemia is very serious, complications due to internal swelling are a possibility *(Rhesus Disease—Symptoms,* 2017).

In times of pregnancy and blood loss, individuals may have anaemia, due to the decrease of iron in the body (*Iron Deficiency Anaemia,* 2017).

In order to be able to increase iron levels in adults, two modes of action are possible (*Iron Deficiency Anaemia*, 2017). One is the consumption and intake of foods with high iron. The second is to contact your family doctor or general practitioner and discuss if iron tablets taken orally are a viable option (*Iron Deficiency Anaemi*a, 2017). Important indicators of reduced iron levels can be fatigue, absence of energy, paler skin, and heart palpitations (*Iron Deficiency Anaemia*, 2017). For the newborn it may be necessary to implement blood transfusion to resolve the anaemia (Dean, 2005).

The following are other common symptoms of Rh disease in newborns: heightened heart rate, faster breathing, lacking energy, skin swelling, and a big abdomen (*Rh Disease—Health Encyclopedia—University of Rochester Medical Center*, n.d.).

Not only is it important to keep an eye out for symptoms, but it is also equally significant to look out for common indicators of Rh disease. The first is the colour of the newborn's skin. If it is yellow, including the whites of the eye, this could indicate jaundice (*Rhesus Disease—Symptoms*, 2017). Jaundice in newborns occur due to an increased level of bilirubin and usually occurs in infants that were delivered before the 38-week mark (*Infant Jaundice—Symptoms and Causes*, n.d.). Additionally, the liver of infants have yet to fully develop and is unable to remove the excessive amounts of bilirubin from the bloodstream (*Infant Jaundice—Symptoms and Causes*, n.d.)

It is important to emphasize that if this disease is left untreated, it can lead to serious complications such as brain damage, deafness, learning difficulties, blindness and stillbirths (*Rhesus Disease*, 2017). That is why there needs to be a focus on prevention and testing of these diseases to begin the treatment process.

Coombs test is a process developed in order to determine if there is incompatibility among the fetus and mother (Dean, 2005). The naming of this testing is derived from Robin Coombs, an immunologist who established the process of detection of antibodies for Rh disease (Dean, 2005). The fundamental idea is to utilize antibodies that connect to the anti-D antibodies (Dean, 2005).This is to aid in the detection of hemolytic disease of the newborn by identifying specific antibodies like the anti-Rh IgG, or Immunoglobulin G, which is an antibody (Dean, 2005).

There are two types of Coombs test, one is direct and it is useful to make a diagnosis of hemolytic disease of the newborn (Dean, 2005). Second is the indirect Coombs test, and its main focus is prevention of hemolytic disease of the newborn (Dean, 2005).

The direct Coombs test focuses on determining if there are antibodies on red blood cells of the fetus, in particular, if anti-D antibodies from the mother are connected to the fetal cells (Dean, 2005). The first step is to take a small amount of red blood cells from the fetus and to remove any connected antibodies. This is done by putting the red blood cells through a wash (Dean, 2005). The next step is to add antibodies onto the red blood cells which clump together and bind to anti-D antibodies (Dean, 2005).

For the indirect Coombs test, it is necessary to locate the presence of anti-D antibodies in serum from the mother (Dean, 2005). This is done before the red blood cells of the fetus have been destroyed (Dean, 2005). Rh-positive red blood cells are mixed with the mother's serum, followed by a wash (Dean, 2005). With the addition of antibodies to this mixture, the goal is to determine if antibodies of the mother are binded (Dean, 2005). This is to determine whether the mother has become sensitized (Dean, 2005). Rh sensitization is the process of exposure of Rh-positive and Rh-negative red blood cells between the fetus and the mother (*Rh Disease—Health Encyclopedia—University of Rochester Medical Center*, n.d.). This leads to an immune system response and results in the mother producing antibodies to destroy fetal blood cells. (*Rh Disease—Health Encyclopedia—University of Rochester Medical Center*, n.d.) Therefore through the Coombs test parents have more information provided to understand the prevention and diagnosis of the disease.

If diagnosis is positive through testing there are treatments that can be applied to preventing hemolytic disease of the newborn (Dean, 2005). The first step is to find out whether the mother has the Rh factor present through performing a blood test (Dean, 2005). The second test is to determine uncommon antibodies absence or presence and this can be done from intake of mother's serum (Dean, 2005).

The second step is determining whether the mother has been sensitized, and this can be done via the indirect coombs test (Dean, 2005). The lack of anti-D on the mother's serum is associated with not being sensitized to the D antigen (Dean, 2005). Administration of the injection of anti-D Ig is given to mothers who are unsensitized and the purpose is to decrease the risk of sensitization in the future (Dean, 2005). Mothers can be injected a series of doses at 28 weeks, 24 weeks, and a couple weeks prior to labor (Dean, 2005). The last dosage can be administered is after birth (Dean, 2005).

If, during the second step, the mother is deemed as sensitized, information of the Rh status of the fetus must be obtained (Dean, 2005). In order to receive a sample from the fetus and determine blood type, fetal cells are obtained via the umbilical cord or amniotic fluid (Dean, 2005). Genetically speaking, the chances the fetus will be positive is determined by the father in reference to the D allele (Dean, 2005). Heterozygous means different forms of the D allele are present and homozygous refers to the same form of the D allele (Dean, 2005). The fetus will be positive, dependent that the father is homozygous (Dean, 2005). On the other hand, there is a 50% chance that the fetus is positive, dependent on the father being heterozygous (Dean, 2005). If the fetus is deemed Rh positive, this means indications of hemolytic disease of the newborn will be monitored through ultrasounds and the mother's serum anti-D amount will be considered (Dean, 2005).

For preventative mechanisms to be effective, it is fundamental to know what population is at risk for Rh disease. Particularly, pregnant women who are Rh negative and the father who happen to be Rh positive have an increased risk for this condition for the fetus to be impacted (*Rh Disease—Health Encyclopedia—University of Rochester Medical Center,* n.d.). Additionally, risk of Rh disease increases if the woman has been previously pregnant (*Rh Disease—Health Encyclopedia—University of Rochester Medical Center,* n.d.). The risk associated with one's first pregnancy is none as long as there is no previous Rh sensitization (*Rh Disease—Health Encyclopedia—University of Rochester Medical Center,* n.d.).

Preventative medicine and treatment are essential components in the management of Rh disease. Additionally, to have a larger perspective on Rh disease and understand how many infants and newborns are impacted by this condition, it is imperative to focus on the mortality and morbidity rates. Medicine and treatment have limitations as many individuals face barriers in terms of accessibility to adequate health care. It is fundamental to determine the barriers of inaccessibility which will be discussed in the following chapters.

CHAPTER 5

Why is RH Disease Worth Investigating?

Written By **Samira Sunderji**

T HIS CHAPTER WILL FOCUS on the mortality rates of neonates diagnosed with Rh disease and will further discuss its associated diseases and illnesses. Additionally, this chapter will discuss the shortfalls of global healthcare in regard to the prevention and treatment of Rh disease, while also discussing the successes of medical advancements and the role of non-profit organizations that aim to eradicate this fatal disease.

During pregnancy, maternal antibodies are transported across the placenta (the organ that nourishes the growing fetus) over its placental barrier and enter the fetal blood circulation. This process is crucial to fetal growth and development as neonates (newborns) possess a primitive immune system that requires ample time to develop outside of the womb (Dean, 2005). The continuing presence of maternal antibodies during postnatal development (the growth and maturation period post birth) ensures that the neonate survives while its immune system matures (Dean, 2005). This is a vital, natural process which is especially of concern if there is an incompatibility of the Rh blood group between the mother and the fetus, as the added maternal protection will specifically target fetal red blood cells (RBCs), also known as erythrocytes. (Dean, 2005).

Rhesus (Rh) incompatibility between maternal and fetal Rh blood types was a major cause of fetal and neonatal morbidity and mortality, as well as long-term disability (Pegoraro, 2020). As stated previously, this incompatibility is due to the crossing of Rh negative maternal blood with Rh positive fetal blood. The result is a production of maternal Rh antibodies (immunoglobulin G (IgG) antibodies) and subsequent damage to fetal red blood cells, which can occur in utero and has the possibility of continuing postnatally outside of the womb. This process causes maternal Rh sensitization. The most common way the crossing between maternal Rh negative blood and fetal Rh positive blood occurs is through delivery (vaginal or C-section). However, other methods include miscarriages, trauma (slips and falls), and invasive procedures such as amniocentesis, where amniotic fluid surrounding the fetus is extracted for testing and treatment procedures (Costumbrado et al., 2020).

As it takes time for mothers to develop RhD antibodies after being exposed to fetal Rh positive blood, first pregnancies and first-born fetuses are usually not affected. However, if a mother is exposed to Rh negative blood at any stage of the first pregnancy or even during delivery, Rh sensitization will occur and has the possibility of affecting subsequent pregnancies. The mother's immune response will react to the Rh factor in fetal blood and produce antibodies to destroy fetal red blood cells. The formation of maternal antibodies in response to fetal Rh antigens is called isoimmunization (Nasser & Webhe, 2020).

The damage to fetal erythrocytes (red blood cells) leads to the process of hemolysis, defined as the breakdown of fetal red blood cells and subsequent release of bilirubin, a yellow compound that arises from said breakdown. The buildup of bilirubin can lead to jaundice, a condition in which the skin, whites of the eyes, and mucous membranes turn yellow. A progressive buildup of bilirubin in the blood (formally known as hyperbilirubinemia) can spread to fetal brain tissues and develop into kernicterus, a rare type of brain damage that occurs in a newborn with severe jaundice caused by excessive bilirubin (Pegoraro, 2020).

Kernicterus affects specific regions of the brain including the basal ganglia (which has a role in motor learning, executive functions, and emotions), the hippocampus (which has a role in learning and memory), geniculate bodies (which have a role in auditory attention), and cranial nerve nuclei (which have a role in sensory inputs and motor outputs) (Hamza, 2019). Kernicterus manifests in 3 separate phases. Phase 1 is defined by a decrease in fetal alertness and decreased muscle tone (hypotonia), which both lead to fatigue, lack of energy, and poor feeding habits. Phase 2 is described as a phase of increased muscle tone (hypertonia) of the extensor muscles found in the upper and lower limbs. However, the increased muscle tone leads to spasticity, where the limb muscles become stiff, and is indicative of abnormal muscle tightness. Progression to phase 2 from phase 1 is an indication that the fetus will have long-term neurological deficits via seizures. Phase 3 is characterized by hypotonia. Further research of kernicterus has indicated a fourth phase that occurs later in infancy and includes relatively permanent signs of extrapyramidal cerebral palsy (Praagh, 1961). This specific type of cerebral palsy has symptoms of abnormal movement patterns, abnormal levels of muscle tone leading to stiffness of limbs, abnormal postural control and a decrease in coordination (Menkes & Curran, 1994). Recent data from the United Kingdom and Canada from 2020 suggests that kernicterus occurs in 1 to 2 in 100,000 live births (Hamza, 2019). The risk of development heightens with increasing buildup of bilirubin in fetal blood. This increase is associated with extremely high risks of irreversible damages as specified earlier.

The breakdown of erythrocytes in the context of Rh disease is formally known as erythroblastosis fetalis or Hemolytic disease of the fetus and newborn (HDN). This disease leads to a lack of healthy red blood cells in fetal circulation to adequately deliver oxygen to bodily tissues, commonly referred to as anemia. Fetal anemia in the context of HDN and Rh disease can lead to extreme heart failure. This is because the fetal heart begins to forcefully pump faster to counter the loss of red blood cells in order to keep up with fetal oxygen demands, which are higher in comparison to those of adults. This is formally known as high-output cardiac failure or myocardial ischemia (Nasser & Webhe, 2020). If left untreated, it can result in premature death (The Regents of the University of California, 2013). Fetal anemia may progress to become severe and life-threatening and leads to fluid accumulation in two or more tissues of the body. This condition is known as hydrops fetalis–where the myocardium (the muscle tissue in the heart) becomes dysfunctional as it has a decreased ability to pump out blood, and this results in swelling (edema), a buildup of fluids (effusions), and increased pressure in the infant's body. (Nasser & Webhe, 2020). Although fluid buildup can occur anywhere in the fetal body, it most often occurs in the abdomen, around the heart and lungs, or under the skin. Outcomes for hydrops fetalis vary greatly based on the gestational age at birth (calculated from the first day of a woman's menstrual cycle) and blood protein levels of the fetus; the complexity of this disease consequently allows for a wide range of mortality (Hamdan, 2017).

Before 1945, approximately 50% of all fetuses born with hemolytic disease of various etiologies, including Rh disease, died of kernicterus or hydrops fetalis (Pegoraro, 2020). In simple terms, Rh disease, in its most severe forms, has the possibility of causing death in utero, stillbirths, or early neonatal death. However, the discovery and development of IgG anti-Rh(D) immunoglobulin or Rho(D) immunoglobulin (RhIG), a neutralizer of Rh positive antigens, was created to prevent the production of maternal Rh antibodies. This has been a major medical achievement and has ultimately reduced the widespread occurrence of Rh disease, particularly in developed countries (Costumbrado, 2020). This preventative method consists of anti-RhD antibodies that target Rh-positive red blood cells in order to prevent maternal sensitization (Costumbrado et al., 2020). Further information on the treatment of Rh disease will be discussed in chapter 9.

From a clinical perspective, the Rhesus blood group system is arguably the most important protein-based blood grouping system, following the

ABO blood grouping system (Flegel, 2007). This is due to its role in understanding and addressing Rh disease and HDN. The first Rhesus gene (the RHCE gene) was discovered in 1990. Two years later, the RhD gene was discovered. Although the Rhesus system is comprised of at least 49 distinct antigens, the discovery and clinical understanding of the presence or absence of the RhD antigen on red blood cells has allowed for a plethora of research experiments and studies to be completed. This has ultimately led to major scientific advances and achievements in medical research, including the development of preventative methods such as anti-D immunoglobulin, as previously stated (Flegel, 2007).

Advancements in Rh disease research allow for the understanding of the disease's various underlying pathophysiological mechanisms. In simpler terms, it allows for researchers to understand the functional changes within the body that accompany the development and progression of Rh disease. Through investigative research, healthcare professionals can be more aware of this disease and, consequently, better care for their patients during pre, peri and postnatal care. To prevent Rh disease from occuring, screening for Rh isoimmunization via blood grouping and crossmatching has become a mandatory practice in Western countries (Agarwal, 2014). This is also known as an Rh factor blood test. If the maternal blood is found to be Rh-D positive, no further testing is required as there is no chance for Rh sensitization and Rh disease. However, if a woman is found to be Rh negative, the case is managed as an isoimmunized pregnancy (Agarwal, 2014). Furthermore, if the test procures an Rh negative result, the paternal blood is also tested in order to determine the Rh status. A high level of concern will only arise if the paternal blood results show Rh positive blood. (Taylor, 2021).

From an epidemiological perspective, those of Caucaisan (North American and European) descent have a higher rate of Rh-negativity (15% to 17%) compared to those of African (4% to 8%) or Asian descent (0.1% to 0.3%) (Costumbrado et al., 2020). As of November 2020, the prevalence of Rh disease is estimated to be 276 per 100,000 live births, as stated in chapter 5 (Costumbrado et al., 2020). Specifically in developed countries (the Western world), the prevalence of Rh disease has been reduced to 2.5 per 100,000 live births (Costumbrado et al., 2020). This gap in prevalence rates between developed and developing countries is attributed to the difference in quality of perinatal and neonatal care in high risk pregnancy cases. A recent study from Columbia University's Irving Medical Centre details how only half of all pregnant women world-wide who are at risk of developing Rh sensitization receive treatment (Columbia University Irving Medical Center, 2020). This investigation began with estimating the annual number of pregnancies worldwide that involve Rh-negative mothers and Rh-positive fetuses. The number of doses of Rho(D) immunoglobulin required to treat the aforementioned women with high-risk Rh pregnancies was calculated. The results were contrasted against the actual number of doses administered globally. The study conclusively found that an annual worldwide gap of 2.5 million doses of Rho(D) immunoglobulin persists today. This is below the minimum recommended threshold for preventing Rh disease. The largest shortfalls for treatment occur in regions of South Asia and Sub-Saharan Africa (Columbia University Irving Medical Center, 2020). The burden of Rh disease in lower-income and developing countries continues to adversely affect fetal mortality rates. A variety of factors influence the high incidents of neonatal deaths including (but not limited to) lack of awareness, inadequate preventative methods, and limited availability to treatment and therapies (Columbia University Irving Medical Center, 2020). These factors are discussed in greater detail in Chapter 8. It is through these scientific investigations that healthcare professionals can gain a deeper level of understanding of Rh disease treatment and can better address these gaps on a regional level, where aid is immediately required.

These findings provoked an international conversation on how medical professionals can best support developing countries in order to reduce neonatal deaths and complications from Rh disease. An international group of collaborators from various medical fields such as obstetrics and gynecology, pediatrics, and neonatology established the Worldwide Initiative Rh Disease Eradication in 2019 (WIRhE) (Columbia University Irving Medical Center, 2020). The WIRhE is a non-profit organization comprised of physicians, scientists, epidemiologists, global health advocates, and industrial partners from around the world who are dedicated towards educating and empowering mothers and families with the goal of one day eradicating Rh disease (WIRhE, 2020). The foundational principles of this organization are encouraging ongoing life-saving projects, enabling healthcare workers to care for mothers and babies via appropriate tools and guidelines, and empowering Rh-positive mothers and families by providing them with foundational information about Rh disease and its prevention (WIRhE, 2020). The WIRhE actively works with other organization such as The International Federation of Gynecology and Obstetrics and the International Confederation of Midwives to review previous research in regards to the usage of anti-Rh(D) immunoglobulin treatment and propose adjusted dosage measurements for different stages and risk factors of Rh disease based on screening tests (Visser et al., 2020). More information on the Worldwide Initiative Rh Disease Eradication and their projects will be thoroughly discussed in chapter 7.Overall, these initiatives shed light on how professionals from various disciplines of medicine and global advocacy are beginning to close (or at least reduce) the gaps in accessing essential medical care and thus, decrease the inequalities within the global healthcare system, particularly of those in developing countries.

Conducting scientific research is a vital component in developing technologies to reduce worldwide health inequities and modernize contemporary forms of medicine in the hopes of eradicating diseases and improving overall quality of life. In the context of Rh disease, the aforementioned advancements of medicine range from deepening our understanding of the Rh factor blood grouping system, to conducting research that investigates the harms of Rh disease on fetuses and neonates. These advancements in research and knowledge allows for reflection on past and present science, and can facilitate next steps in research that focus on prevention and treatment. Healthcare professionals can use this knowledge to care for patients who are at high risk for developing Rh sensitization and disease. This is the primary reason why the prevalence of Rh disease in fetuses and neonates has significantly reduced in developed countries–it is attributable to the continued efforts of professionals from various medical disciplines who have worked tirelessly to make such advancements possible. However, knowledge translation from field investigations to published research studies does not have to stop there. Science is valued by societies across the globe as the application of scientific knowledge aims to satisfy many basic human needs and improve living standards (Rull, 2014). Specifically, science education and communication to the general public is an important application of scientific research that empowers everyone to better care for themselves and others. For those who are unable to access this information, organizations such as the WIRhE are actively trying to address such problems in order to provide care for all, regardless of socioeconomic status, age, gender, and geographical location. Therefore, continued scientific research investigations in the field of Rh disease will aim to spread awareness by providing ample knowledge to the general public on the disease itself, and will allow for healthcare professionals to adequately and successfully care for all mothers and fetuses who are at risk of developing Rh disease.

More information on the science behind the discovery of Rh disease and its pathophysiology will be discussed in the following chapter with a focus on genetics and screening tests.

CHAPTER 6

What science is involved in studying Rh disease?

*Written By **Si Cong (Sam) Zhang***

A S HAS BEEN STATED IN previous chapters, Rh disease is the most common type of Hemolytic Disease of the Fetus and Newborn (HDFN). As suggested by its name, HDFN is a category of diseases that is characterized by the destruction(-lytic) of the red blood cells (hemo-) in the fetus. The cause of HDFN is an inappropriate immune response by the mother against the fetal red blood cells (RBC). This immune response takes the form of IgG antibodies produced by the mother which attack the fetal RBCs, destroying them rapidly (Bussel & Despotovic, 2014). Antigens are the specific characteristics of the fetal cells which the antibody recognizes and attacks, the different types of antigen expressed on the fetal RBCs results in different types of HDFN (Berg et al., 2002). Several different types of HDFN exist, including ABO, anti-RhD, anti-RhE, anti-Rhc, anti-Rhe, anti-RhC, anti-Kell, and combinations of others. The anti-RhD type is the most common type of HDFN, and is also known as Rh disease (Fan et al., 2014). It is important to understand the mechanism behind Rh disease in order to understand what scientific techniques are used to study it and why we use them.

To better understand these mechanisms, it is helpful to think about how a mother's body usually interacts with the fetus in her womb. During fertilization, genetic information from both parents is combined into an embryo which will develop into a fetus. It is important to recognize that both paternal (from the father) and maternal (from the mother) genomes are present within the embryo. As the embryo develops, a placenta is formed, which allows the exchange of nutrients between the embryo and the mother. For the most part, the blood of the fetus and the mother are kept in separate circulations, but sometimes a fetomaternal hemorrhage (FMH) occurs. This is when fetal RBCs cross into the mother's blood due to damage to the placenta (Krywko et al., 2021). Normally this is non-problematic (Solomonia et al., 2012) as the mother's immune system recognizes the fetal cells as one of their own. Sometimes, however, an inappropriate immune response occurs. What causes this inappropriate response is when the mother's immune system recognizes the fetal cells as foreign (isoimmunity/alloimmunity) (Katz et al., 1984).

In this sequence of events, there are factors from across the disciplines of biology, which should be addressed. First, it is important to answer the most fundamental question: "How do cells know what their enemies are?" This question underlies all immunity-related diseases, and one would not be able to continue without a clear understanding. Second, it is important to understand the effect of blood type including the Rhesus protein on the immune system. Third, a basic knowledge of genetic inheritance is necessary to understand the genetic basis of Rh disease. Lastly, some understanding of human anatomy isrequired, especially knowledge of the placenta.

The human immune system is a powerful weapon developed over thousands of years of evolution. It consists of 2 major parts: innate immunity and adaptive immunity. Innate immunity is the non-specific branch of the immune system; it does not target any specific pathogen, but instead, causes a general, effective response. The adaptive immune system, on the other hand, is very effective against specific antigens and has a lasting "memory" of previous infections. Adaptive immunity is responsible for vaccines and long-term immunity, but it is also the culprit behind Rh disease (The Innate and Adaptive Immune Systems, 2020).

When the cells responsible for recognizing antigens (called antigen-presenting cells) are produced in the thymus (an organ located just below your neck), they are checked for their ability to bind to antigens found on the body's own cells. Evidently, if an antigen-presenting cell did bind to its own cells, then it would recognize its own organs and tissues as foreign and summon other cells to attack the body's own organs. That's not wanted, so these are normally removed from the pool of potential antigen-presenting cells. When the antigen-presenting cells do recognize an antigen, they call for a B cell (an immune cell that produces antibodies). B cells can then produce massive amounts of antibodies which destroy the antigen (Berg et al., 2002).

But what is triggering this immune response in Rh disease? And how can it be proven?

Rh disease is caused by an incompatibility in blood type between the fetus and the mother, but not the ABO blood types one is more familiar with (Rh Incompatibility—NHLBI, Nih, n.d.). Blood type is determined by the presence of A and B proteins on the surface of the red blood cells. Type A blood is positive for the A protein but not the B protein, type B is the opposite, type AB has both proteins, and type O has none. These blood types are determined via hemagglutination. Hemagglutination is simply the clumping of blood when two different blood types are mixed ("Commentary on and Reprint of Landsteiner k, Ueber Agglutinationserscheinungen Normalen Menschlichen Blute [on the Agglutination of Normal Human Blood], in Wiener Klinische Wochenschrift (1901) 14," 2000). This is caused by antibodies for the other blood type binding red blood cells together into clumps. When blood of the same type is mixed, neither person has antibodies targeting the other's red blood cells since they present the same antigen and the RBCs don't clump. Nowadays, blood tests use purified antibodies for each of these antigens.

However, some may know that there is also a positive or negative associated with each of the four blood types, such as A+ and A-. The positive and negative indicate the presence of the Rhesus protein. This was not originally known since most people have the Rhesus protein, and thus no clumps formed when two samples of the same ABO blood types are mixed. However, a minority of the population lacks the Rhesus protein, and will therefore develop antibodies targeting the Rhesus protein (Dean, 2005). Hemagglutination is also performed here to test for the presence of the Rhesus protein. If blood clumps in the presence of Rhesus protein antibodies, then the blood is Rh-positive (Wiener, 1952).

Now, imagine if there were some kind of injury, either caused by a medical procedure, an accident, or simply a tear during childbirth and a tiny bit of the fetal Rh+ blood enters the bloodstream of the maternal Rh- blood. The immune system cells of the mother detect the Rh antigens on the surface of the fetal RBCs, it considers the fetal RBCs a foreign invader and starts the process of producing antibodies against the Rh antigen (Cortey et al., 2006). One specific type of antibody, the IgG antibody is able to pass through the placental barrier, from the mother to the fetus. Normally, this is intended to immunize the newborn against pathogens for the first few months of its life by storing these maternal antibodies in the blood of the infant. This way, if an infection occurs, the maternal antibodies can contribute to fighting off infections (Charles A Janeway et al., 2001). However, if the mother's immune system produces IgG antibodies that target the fetal RBCs and these antibodies pass through the placental barrier, they would destroy the RBCs within the fetus (Bussel & Despotovic, 2014).

While the determination of Rh disease is in the field of immunology, why the child is Rh positive or Rh negative can only be determined by genetics. Every human carries two copies of the same chromosome, and thus two copies of the same gene 1. A minority of the population carries the Rh- version of the gene, and the majority of the population carries the Rh+ version of the gene. The Rh+ version is dominant over the Rh- version, meaning if a person has 1 copy of Rh- and Rh+, their blood type will still be Rh+. An Rh- blood type can only occur when someone has the Rh- version on both copies of the chromosomes (Flegel, 2007).

When fertilization occurs, one of the two copies from both parents is selected at random and passed on to the child. Therefore the child will have one copy from each parent, and the potential versions of the Rh gene the child possesses can be represented graphically using a "Punnett square".

In a Punnett square, the genetic composition of the parents is placed on either axis, each column or row represents one version of the gene that the parent possesses, and the potential genetic composition of the child can be found where the columns and rows intersect. In this case, we are only considering the possibilities where the mother is Rh- because that is one of the requirements for Rh disease.

If the father also has 2 copies of the Rh- version of the gene, the child will 100% be Rh- as well. There is a 0% chance of Rh disease occurring if the blood of the mother and fetus mixes.

If the father also has copies of both versions of the gene, the child will have a 50% of being Rh- and a 50% chance of being Rh+. There is a 50% chance of Rh disease occurring if the blood of the mother and the fetus mixes.

Father

		+	-
Mother	-	- +	- -
	-	- +	- -

If the father also has two copies of the Rh+ versions of the gene, the child will have a 100% chance of being Rh+. 100% chance of Rh disease occurring if the blood of the mother and fetus mixes ("Can Two Rh-Positive Parents Have an Rh-Negative Child?", 2018).

Father

		+	+
Mother	-	- +	- +
	-	- +	- +

This is why usually before a planned pregnancy, or immediately after conception, doctors may recommend that the parents take a blood test. The blood test will test for various diseases which can be passed from mother to child such as HIV, but also the blood type in cases of Rh disease. If there is the possibility of Rh disease occurring, the parents can be warned and appropriate treatments prepared ahead of time (Rhesus Disease, 2017). See chapter 9 for the different treatments used for Rh disease.

One of the treatments discussed is Rh immune globulin (RhIG). The specific effects of the treatment and effectiveness can be found in chapter 9. Simply put, it is using purified antibodies against the Rh antigen coming from the fetus. Acting by an identical mechanism as antibodies produced if the mother's immune system were activated, these antibodies bind to any fetal red blood cells which may have entered the mother's circulatory system and destroys them before the mother's immune system can be activated (*Rho(D) Immune Globulin Monograph for Professionals*, 2021).

While this explanation of the activation of the maternal immune system sounds plausible and makes perfect sense, it is entirely dependent on the fact that the fetal blood does, in fact, mix with the maternal blood. To prove that such an event occurs before the onset of Rh disease, scientists have developed very elegant techniques for identifying if fetal blood is present and the number of fetal RBCs in maternal blood. The Rosette test is a screening test used to test if fetal blood is present, and if the result is positive, then the amount present can be quantified by one of two methods (Nester et al., 2018). The older method is called the "Kleihauer Betke Test" (Krywko et al., 2021) and the newer method is called "flow cytometry" (Kennedy et al., 2003).

The rosette test is conducted on an RhD- mother with an RhD+ child to determine if fetal RhD+ cells are present in maternal blood. The rosette test is a qualitative test, meaning that the result of the test is not a definitive number but instead a category such as "yes" or "no". It is used as a screening test because of its relative simplicity and speed (Van Buren, 2019). The principle behind the rosette test is the same antibody-antigen binding principle as described previously. A sample of the maternal blood is mixed with anti-RhD antibodies which will bind to any RhD+ fetal blood cells in the blood. Then red indicator RhD+ RBCs will be added, and become stuck to the RhD+ fetal cell. Then the result can be plated and viewed under a microscope. Because normal unstained RBCs will appear near-transparent under a microscope, it is very easy to find any red indicator RBCs. The red indicator RBCs will form a clump with several indicator RBCs stuck to the sides of a fetal cell, resembling the petals of a flower, hence the name "rosette test" (Lee & Kaufman, 2011).

While the rosette test is a cost-effective and rapid solution, it has significant limitations. The most obvious is the fact that one is unable to determine the severity of FMH as one can't determine the amount of fetal blood present in the sample. In order for the doctor to prescribe the appropriate amount of RhIG, the amount of fetal blood is required. In addition, the rosette test only works when the mother is RhD- and the child is RhD+. It is sufficient for use in addressing Rh disease but ineffective for other kinds of FMH. In situations where more information is needed, the two quantitative tests can be performed.

The Kleihauer Betke "KB" Test also known as the Kleihauer Betke stain, Kleihauer test or acid elution test, is the most commonly used test to quantify FMH in the United States (Lee & Kaufman, 2011). The test takes advantage of the different forms of hemoglobin between maternal RBCs and fetal RBCs. The fetal form of hemoglobin HbF is much more resistant to acid than the adult form HbA. Thus, a blood smear is exposed to an acid solution, after which the HbA is removed but the HbF remains intact. Then the cells are stained using erythrosin B, a dye that binds to HbF in the fetal cells, allowing them to be counted. The percentage of fetal cells to maternal cells can then be calculated (Krywko et al., 2021).

The downsides of the KB test are that it is highly labour intensive as the number of cells must be counted, but this may change in the future as computers may be able to automate this process. In addition, the KB test tends to overestimate the number of fetal cells if the mother has certain conditions such as sickle cell anemia or b-thalassemia (Lee &

Kaufman, 2011).

A newer technique involving flow cytometry is also now being used more and more, as it is more accurate, more efficient, and more reproducible (Lee & Kaufman, 2011). Because flow cytometry gives a lower and more accurate measure of the amount of fetal blood present, patients can receive a lower dose of RhIG (Van Buren, 2019). To count the number of cells using flow cytometry, the samples of RBCs are first mixed with fluorescent antibodies. These antibodies attach themselves to the target fetal cells and make them fluorescent. Then the cells are passed through an excitation beam one at a time, and when the fluorescent cells are hit by the beam, they fluoresce and can be detected. The number of excitations is counted and the number of fetal cells can be deduced. In addition, flow cytometry has the added benefit of having two different kinds of antibodies which can be used, anti-D or anti-HbF. This way, it is possible to detect fetal cells even if they are not Rh-positive (Kennedy et al., 2003).

Characteristic of all scientific endeavours, most of the techniques used to study Rh disease described in this chapter can also be applied to a wide range of other medical purposes. For example, rosetting is also used to identify other blood cells such as T cells, and fluorescent-labelled antibodies are also used to visualize certain organelles in microscopy. It is therefore also extremely important that one understands that science is a cumulative effort by many individuals across multiple generations, building on the works of others. While today we look back and can easily understand the principles of antigens, antibodies, and their relationship with blood typing, this information was not yet clear to Landsteiner when he first described the interactions between blood types in his paper "Ueber Agglutinationserscheinungen normalen menschlichen Blute" published in 1901. And, of course, it would have been impossible for him and Alexander S. Wiener to have discovered Rh blood types in 1937 if he did not discover blood types some 30 years ago. When one imagines a brighter tomorrow with better and faster techniques, it is also important that one remembers the steps we are taking to get there. That's why it would be of great interest for many readers to read about the early research done if they want a more whole image of the medical research landscape.

In the next chapter, the recent discoveries about Rh disease will be discussed in detail.

CHAPTER 7

What have We Learned About RH Disease in Recent Medical History?

*Written By **Anusha Mappanasingam***

IN CHAPTER 2, WE DISCUSSED the discovery of Rh disease and have presented the necessity in investigating the disease and the science behind it in chapters 5 and 6 respectively. From the information presented and discussed, the tremendous impact that the research conducted has on the prevalence of Rh disease in various communities becomes obvious: the prevalence rates of Rh disease has been lowered significantly. This impact on populations affected by Rh disease is also primarily due to prevention methods that have surfaced for women with RhD negative blood; these prevention methods will be discussed further in chapter 9. While the research obtained has also ensured the widespread knowledge of Rh disease amongst most communities and has assisted in making prevention methods for Rh disease well-known and accessible for the developed part of the world, efforts are continuously made by researchers and clinicians to expand on the knowledge we have thus far obtained. In this chapter, the various findings that have been discovered and learned regarding Rh disease in recent medical history will be presented and discussed. Specifically, we will briefly consider the prominent research conducted regarding Rh disease, as well as explore specifics with regards to the inspirations these discoveries have provided for current research and education in Rh disease. Lastly, we will conclude with the recent specific discoveries made regarding the global unequal distribution of educational resources and preventative measures for Rh disease

Surprisingly enough, there is actually minimal significant research done on Rh disease in the last couple of years. Although this might suggest that researchers and clinicians lack interest in furthering research in Rh disease, or fail to notice its importance, it is important to highlight that this is actually not the case. Most of the prominent research regarding Rh disease has actually taken place decades ago. One of our first insights into this disease was when Dr. Karl Landsteiner and Dr. Alexander S. Wiener discovered the Rh factors in the 1940s (Landsteiner & Wiener, 1941). From that point on many crucial discoveries were made regarding transfusions and preventative measures, with many contributions coming from Canada. More details about the historical discovery of Rh disease in the mid-twentieth century are presented in chapter 2, while details about preventative measures and their efficiency can be found in chapter 9.

Regardless of the radio silence around Rh disease, these historical moments of discovery from the past have begun to inspire specific avenues of research. While the future research potential of Rh disease will be discussed in more detail in chapter 11, let us briefly discuss some of the fairly new discoveries that have been made in the recent decades. One of these recent discoveries is prenatal genotyping of fetal blood groups (Stockman, 2001). This technique uses sources including amniotic fluid or fetal cells in the mother's blood to determine if there is a chance for the newborn to get hemolytic disease, whose applications are further discussed in chapter 3 (Stockman, 2001). One of the research avenues that are currently being considered is incorporating more molecular analysis to determine why some Rh negative women are more susceptible to sensitization. (Stockman, 2001). Another recent development is the realization of late hyporegenerative anemia—a form of anemia associated with hemolytic disease—in newborns (Stockman,

2001). Specifically, it has been determined that it is the limited frequency of transfusions involving the removal of the mother's antibody occurring after birth is what causes this late anemia; they have moved to perform intravascular transfusions before birth (Stockman, 2001). The limited postpartum transfusions occurring causes late anemia because these infants begin to have seen an increase in amounts of their mother's antibodies (Stockman, 2001). This is dangerous as these antibodies remove red blood cells that are formed after childbirth (Stockman, 2001). Nowadays, clinicians use recombinant erythropoietin—erythropoietin being a concept that will be briefly covered in chapter 9—to stop late hyporegenerative anemia or to reduce the number of transfusions that newborns undergo (Stockman, 2001).

From what we've discussed so far, one might conclude that the majority of the children are safe from Rh disease: the combined efforts of the knowledge obtained decades ago, the institutes advocating for Rh disease education and research, and the preventative measures for mothers promoted and practiced today are significant and have been proven to work. However, considering Rh disease from a global perspective has inspired researchers to shift the focus of their research in order to analyze the impact of Rh disease in developing countries. This has led to the discovery that the conclusion of lower susceptibility rates to Rh disease is an inaccurate interpretation of the current data. In recent history, researchers have discovered that while the prevalence of Rh disease is significantly low in developed countries, it continues to exist as a relevant issue in developing countries around the world (Bhutani et al., 2013). An analysis by researchers across the world was made in 2010 with a study discussing the prevalence of Rh disease and extreme jaundice in newborns on regional and global scales (Bhutani et al., 2013). Through the analysis of literature and the collection of country-specific data, researchers were able to use a three-step compartmental modeling approach that could digest country-specific information to determine prevalence rates of Rh disease (Bhutani et al., 2013). They proposed an estimate of 373 300 babies being affected by Rh disease in 2010 on a global scale (Bhutani et al., 2013). While the worldwide prevalence for Rh disease was found to be 276 for every 100 000 live births, it is when comparing the region-specific outcomes to global values that we are confronted with the undeniable truth. Rh disease continues to persist in developing countries at an alarming rate (Bhutani et al., 2013). When considering the statistics obtained in the study, it becomes apparent that the prevalence of Rh disease in specific regions is significantly higher than the 276/100 000 obtained to represent global values (Bhutani et al., 2013). In South Asia, sub-Saharan Africa, and Eastern Europe/ Central Asia, their models estimates a prevalence rate of 385, 386, and 529 for every 100 000 live births, respectively; this is nearly a 100/100 000 increase when compared to global values, with the latter facing an increase of approximately 250/100 000 live births (Bhutani et al., 2013). Since many believed that Rh disease was no longer an issue, these prevalence rates that are being uncovered are higher than what many believed. This becomes more evident when we are presented with the prevalence of Rh disease in developed countries: 2.5 for every 100 000 live births (Bhutani et al., 2013). This drastic difference in the frequency of Rh disease thus highlights the possibility that preventative measures for this disease are not actively practiced in developing countries; the reasons why are questions the researchers are trying to address.

While considering the various studies done in different parts of the world, the reasons for Rh disease's continued occurrence in these countries becomes clear: one of the primary causes is a lack of awareness. Generally, the unresolved issue stems from the lack of awareness of the disease itself; this is closely related to the fact that developing countries tend to suffer from a lack of educational resources surrounding matters related to Rh disease. This discovery was made across multiple studies over the recent years. From a 2019 study conducted in Brazil, researchers conducted a survey that targeted neonatologists, pediatricians, nurses, physiotherapists, and other healthcare professionals as their responding audience to discuss their workplace's Rh disease-related practices (Variane & Sant'Anna, 2021). Researchers were able to find that only

66% of individuals who responded were aware of their hospital's or medical centre's policy for Rh disease screening, while 18% worked in institutions that lacked such a policy and 16% were not sure of whether such a policy existed (Variane & Sant'Anna, 2021). Additionally, of the respondents, 44% did not know whether mothers received preventative measures like Rh immunoglobulin (Variane & Sant'Anna, 2021). From these results, researchers were able to identify the presence of significant gaps in knowledge amongst professionals regarding Rh disease policy, Rh disease prevalence, and matters involving preventative treatment (Variane & Sant'Anna, 2021). Interestingly, where this lack of awareness of matters involving Rh disease was derived, they were also able to conclude an obvious lack of publication on Rh disease in Brazil (Variane & Sant'Anna, 2021). While considering this study and comparing it to the prevalence values that were discussed earlier, we are forced to contend with the idea that rather than a lack of access to preventative treatments, it is the lack of recognition and knowledge of the general healthcare systems and policies that cause prevalence rates in developing countries to be significantly higher than the developed world. While the low-income populations of developing countries make the idea of gaining access to preventative treatments a momentous issue that is worthy of consideration, the lack of knowledge needs to be addressed immediately in order to allow global leaders to begin implementing policies that will consider the unequal distribution of Rh disease treatments.

By conducting studies to obtain and analyze statistical evidence reflecting the impact of Rh disease, researchers begin their initiative to make changes on global scales by informing clinicians, policy makers, and other individuals in power about the details regarding the high prevalence of Rh disease in the wake of its known preventability. Specifically, organizations involved in advocating for Rh disease awareness and prevention have taken measures to highlight policy changes they recommend for other healthcare institutions. In 2021, the International Federation of Gynecology and Obstetrics (FIGO) and the International

Confederation of Midwives (ICM) collaborated with the Worldwide Initiative for Rh Disease Eradication (WIRhE) organization to propose new guidelines for preventing Rh disease (Visser et al., 2021). Prior to proposing these guidelines, they presented a summary of the current usage of anti-Rh(D) immunoglobulin to remind individuals of some of the preventative measures that are actively used and are available. Currently, anti-Rh(D) immunoglobulin is actively administered after Rh(D) negative women give birth, during pregnancy, after miscarriages, ectopic pregnancies, amniocentesis, abdominal trauma, and intrauterine fetal death (Visser et al., 2021).

While more details about inconsistencies with anti-Rh(D) immunoglobulin administration can be found in chapter 9, it is crucial to emphasize some notes these organizations conducting the study make toward the effectiveness of anti-Rh(D) immunoglobulin administration in certain cases. One of the cases in question is amniocentesis; most countries ensure that Rh(D) negative pregnant women are given anti-Rh(D) immunoglobulin after undergoing this procedure (Visser et al., 2021). However, this is done despite the lack of evidence present to support this as a beneficial course of treatment (Visser et al., 2021). Additionally, there is also a lack of clarity in the varying doses administered: doses are often offered without sufficient evidence or reasoning to support the amount given (Visser et al., 2021). For example, when administering anti-Rh(D) immunoglobulin after pregnancy, there have been reports recommending doses of 500 IU and some using 1 500 IU, with minimal reasoning offered (Visser et al., 2021). While it is expected that different healthcare systems might implement different dosages, this inconsistency appears to have no reasoning. This can make it harder for developing countries to establish health-care protocols in an effective way. In other scenarios, the ideal dose is unknown. This is the case when administering anti-Rh(D) immunoglobulin for those suffering from abdominal trauma, vaginal bleeding, and fetal death (Visser et al., 2021). By communicating this gap in knowledge, scientists illustrate our need for more research on dosage to prevent Rh disease.

In this study, these organizations propose new guidelines for dosage and prioritization. They recommend three categories for prioritizing treatment: high priority, middle priority, and low priority (Visser et al., 2021). The high priority category includes the cases in which clinicians are determining the Rh factor, as well as the consequent determination of the Rh factor of newborns with Rh(D) negative mothers (Visser et al., 2021). High priority cases also include post-delivery periods, specifically for Rh(D) negative women who have not been synthesized and had just given birth to Rh(D) positive babies (Visser et al., 2021). Also included in this category are recommended doses: a standard 500 IU of anti-Rh(D) immunoglobulin is sufficient, but 1 500 IU can be given if resources of the country permits (Visser et al., 2021). Researchers have defined the middle priority category to include administering anti-Rh(D) immunoglobulin during pregnancy, for miscarriages and ectopic pregnancies, and for abdominal trauma or fetal death, with 1 500 IU, 500 IU, and 500 IU/1 500 IU as respective doses (Visser et al., 2021). Lastly, the low priority section contains administering 500 IU after amniocentesis (Visser et al., 2021). Overall, these new guidelines call for changes in Rh disease policy globally. They emphasize the current need for Rh disease education so preventative measures can be offered efficiently.

Studies like those just discussed have provided valuable information for the public. Since this research is publicly accessible to an extent, members of the public are given the opportunity to educate themselves and others. It also encourages them to proceed with taking up precautions that are necessary with Rh disease. However, these studies are not the only way in which researchers have advocated for Rh disease education and research. Researchers' common goal— to eradicate Rh disease globally has inspired the establishment of multiple organizations. One of these organizations is actually one that contributed to an impactful study that was previously discussed in this chapter. As discussed in chapter 5, the Worldwide Initiative for Rh Disease Eradication (WIRhE) is an international association aiming to globally abolish Rh disease. WIRhE was formed after researchers became aware of the harsh reality of the high prevalence of Rh disease due to a lack of awareness and access to treatment in more than half the world (*WIRhE—Worldwide Initiative for Rh Diseas Eradication*, n.d.). Hoping to tackle this situation directly, on March 29th 2019, WIRhE was formed in Rome; this founding group of scientists and clinicians now work with individuals in varying positions around the world, and have partnered with institutions like the South Central Association of Blood Banks, SickKids, and the International Society of Blood Transfusion to achieve their goals (*WIRhE—Worldwide Initiative for Rh Diseas Eradication*, n.d.). The founder and current executive director, Dr. Steven L. Spitalnik, along with his peers, fights to eliminate Rh disease in developing countries by supporting crucial projects, providing healthcare workers with effective tools to care for families, and empowering Rh negative mothers through education on Rh disease and prevention (*WIRhE—Worldwide Initiative for Rh Diseas Eradication*, n.d.). Asides from studies they have contributed to, such as the one mentioned previously, WIRhE provides a unique approach to ending Rh disease in developing parts of the world; this approach is discussed in chapter 5. Another organization that is currently advocating for Rh disease is the non-profit organization known as the Winnipeg Rh Institute Foundation (*Winnipeg RH Institute Foundation*, n.d.). The founder of this institute, Dr. John Bowman, developed and released the vaccine called WinRho, a treatment for Rh disease, in 1973. It is responsible for saving thousands of newborn lives (*Winnipeg RH Institute Foundation*, n.d.). Today, the Winnipeg Rh Institute Foundation works to advance efforts to improve children's health in two ways: their Rh awards and financial support (*Winnipeg RH Institute Foundation*, n.d.). Since 1992, this foundation has provided around $4.5 million to financially support children's health related research (*Winnipeg RH Institute Foundation*, n.d.). Additionally, the Winnipeg Rh Institute Foundation aims to provide recognition for hard-working individuals through their yearly Rh awards (*Winnipeg RH Institute Foundation*, n.d.). These awards were established in 1973 and given to beginner researchers at the University of Manitoba who demonstrated dedication and promise in their field (*Winnipeg RH Institute Foundation*, n.d.). It is through the efforts of these organizations that researchers and clinicians are able to share their discoveries surrounding Rh disease in developing countries, and encourage individuals to advocate for its eradication.

In conclusion, this chapter aimed to present and evaluate the new findings that were made revolving around Rh disease in recent medical history. It was immediately highlighted that the majority of our prominent work with Rh disease was done decades ago, in the 1940s-1960s. This was followed by a brief look into new research avenues that have been considered in the recent years, including prenatal genotype testing of fetal blood groups and the discovery of late hyporegenerative anemia and its link to transfusions. Readers were then presented with the major Rh disease-related finding of recent years: the continued prevalence of Rh disease in developing countries. Along with this, we looked at the problems associated with the doses of anti-Rh(D) immunoglobulin currently offered, and the recommended changes provided by some Rh disease research groups. Lastly, we had a brief look into some of the current initiatives regarding Rh disease and the impact they aim to have.

Due to the prevalence of Rh disease in developing countries and the nature of the preventative measures in use, researchers and clinicians are eager to expand the depth of their knowledge on Rh disease. In the next chapter, current questions revolving around Rh disease will be presented and contemplated.

CHAPTER 8

What Questions are We Still Asking about RH Disease?

Written By **Rishi Thangarajah**

INTRODUCTION

Since Rh disease was first discovered in 1940, our understanding of the disease has vastly improved. Researchers and clinicians alike now know that Rh disease occurs when anti-D antibodies, produced by a sensitized Rh-negative mother, signal the destruction of red blood cells in her Rh-positive fetus. In previous chapters, the various clinical presentations and medical complications resulting from the hemolytic nature of Rh disease were discussed. In addition to this, in chapter 6, we explored the pathogenesis behind these adverse outcomes associated with Rh disease. The goal of this chapter is to address some of the questions surrounding Rh disease that remain unanswered. Chapter 7 gave you some insight into the issues developing nations have with Rh disease. The remainder of this chapter will supplement that information and build upon your understanding of challenges in treating Rh disease. A holistic approach will be utilized to examine the infrastructural, economical, political and social questions linked to Rh disease.

You might assume that with all this knowledge of Rh disease paired with the application of preventive Rh disease treatments, proven to be effective, that Rh disease has been eradicated. Unfortunately, this is not the case. Worldwide it is estimated that for every 100,000 live births that occur, 276 newborns are affected by Rh disease (Costumbrado, Mansour & Chassemzadeh, 2020). It is expected that approximately half of all untreated newborns with HDN will either develop brain damage or die as a result of Rh disease (Costumbrado, Mansour & Chassemzadeh, 2020). This statistic is truly heartbreaking when you consider the fact that the loss of the lives of these newborns is preventable. Which begs the question; if newborn deaths related to Rh disease are avoidable, why do they still happen?

A TALE OF TWO WORLDS

The answer to this question is complex, convoluted and goes beyond the scope of what we consider to be traditional medical science. Unlike most diseases, the knowledge gaps associated with Rh disease are not related to an unknown signaling pathway or mechanism. Rather, it is the unique interplay between human health and the surrounding environment that creates new questions linked to Rh disease. Previous chapters hinted that certain groups of people within the global population are hit harder by Rh disease than others. Therefore, identifying these vulnerable populations could help determine *"why Rh disease still exists?"*. Imagine if you were tasked with categorizing the human population contained on this planet, what methodology would you employ? You might settle on separating populations based on demographic factors such as age, ethnicity or gender. Alternatively, you may decide to simply group populations together based on geopolitical barriers such as one's nationality. In the subdiscipline of global health, experts in the field opt to divide the population under the broader context of being either a part of the developed or developing world. These overarching terms are used to categorize countries into one of the two "worlds". Think of the developed and developing world like apples and oranges, in that they have similar components, however these components harbour distinct qualities that differentiate them from one another. Developed countries, for instance Canada, typically have a higher human development index, or HDI, value than their developing counterparts (Human

Development Report, 2020). An HDI value takes dimensions like the life expectancy, knowledge and gross domestic product, or GDP, per capita of a country in order to ascertain quality of life in that region (Human Development Report, 2020).

It is imperative to distinguish between the two 'worlds' when aiming to answer the unknown questions surrounding Rh disease. This is because the distribution of Rh disease is disproportional across the globe (Pegoraro et al, 2020). You see, Rh disease has essentially been eradicated within the borders of developed nations (Zipursky, Bhutani & Odame, 2015). In the developed world, for every 100,000 live births, less than 3 newborns are affected by Rh disease (Costumbrado, Mansour & Chassemzadeh, 2020). The prevalence of Rh cases in the developed world is substantially smaller than the worldwide prevalence: 276 newborns affected by Rh disease for every 100,000 live births. Consequently, this means that the estimated amount of cases is skewed by the impact Rh disease has upon the developing world. It is likely that the number of newborns in the developing world affected by Rh disease greatly exceeds current global estimations.

The information above provides us with the answer to our original question of *"why Rh disease still exists?"*. The reason Rh disease still affects newborns on a global scale is because the developing world is struggling to eliminate the disease. Although this answer appears simple, it does little to resolve the remaining questions surrounding Rh disease. If anything it does the opposite by introducing follow-up questions, for instance *"why is the developing world struggling with Rh disease, when preventative treatments exist?"*. Think of the eradication of Rh disease in the developing word as an expedition across the ocean. If we consider 0 newborns affected by Rh disease to be the end goal, then the questions related to Rh disease can be thought of as an iceberg obstructing the route to that destination. At face value, the question appears to be singular and simple enough to answer. However, much like how the majority of an iceberg's mass is hidden beneath the surface of the ocean, a lack of perspective masks increasingly complex follow-up questions. Encounters with tough questions should be anticipated along the journey in eliminating Rh disease worldwide. The developed world is already extremely close to reaching this destination, but the developing world is noticeably lagging behind. In order to reach the "destination", the developing world must address how they will begin to answer these difficult questions. Therefore, instead of asking *"why has Rh disease not been eradicated yet?"*, a better question would be *"how can we reduce the global estimate of newborns affected by Rh disease from 276 per 100,000 live births to 0?"*.

INFRASTRUCTURAL QUESTIONS

The course of action seems quite straightforward based on what has been discussed so far. If Rh disease predominantly affects newborns in the developing world, the optimal course of action to eliminate the disease would be to administer the prophylaxis, or preventative treatment, to Rh negative women residing within the developing world. It is here that we run into our first unanswered question surrounding Rh disease, *"exactly how many women in the developing world are Rh negative?"*. You may have noticed that whenever cases of Rh disease in the developing world are referred to, they are prefaced by terms such as estimation or assumptions. The reasoning behind this being that, the exact burden of Rh disease in the developing world is unknown (Pegoraro et al, 2020). Unlike the developed world that has healthcare databases and systems in place, this is not the situation certain developing countries find themselves in (Al Dahdah, Du Loû & Méadel, 2015). Research reveals that common issues plaguing healthcare institutions in the developing world include a deficiency in the number of healthcare institutions due to limited resources and poor policy planning (Dela Cruz & Ortega-Dela Cruz, 2018).

While this may be true, by adopting a technocentric view, it may be plausible to circumvent this issue. A technocentric view refers to the belief that technology will undoubtedly undergo a requisite level of innovation required to solve issues that arise in the future. For example, smartphones offer a technological solution to the issue of poor healthcare management. Smartphone use in the developing world has actually been increasing since 2013 (Al Dahdah, Du Loû & Méadel, 2015). For every 100 individuals in the developing world, 89 of them have an activated line of communication (Al Dahdah, Du Loû & Méadel, 2015). Using SMS, cloud technology and the flash memory storage contained within a smartphone, it would be possible to create and update a healthcare database without a heavy reliance on healthcare personnel (Al Dahdah, Du Loû & Méadel, 2015). This strategy would likely have to be paired with rapid diagnostic testing for Rh status—a concept that is discussed in chapter 11 in extensive detail—in order to be successful. Fortunately, many non-governmental organizations, or NGOs, have realized the potential benefit mobile health can have on maternal care in developing nations (Al Dahdah, Du Loû & Méadel, 2015). The lack of access to adequate healthcare and supplies was one of the obstacles mentioned regarding the elimination of Rh disease in the developing world (Pegoraro et al, 2020). If demographic data, including the physical geographic distribution of Rh negative women was known, then effective strategies could be implemented to bring humankind closer to the eradication of Rh disease. Instead of having Rh negative women travel in from remote areas to the nearest healthcare facility, temporary clinics in locations within the proximity of Rh-negative clusters could be utilized to administer the treatment to the women that require it.

However, it is important to note that the quality of the developing world's healthcare infrastructure determines how many Rh-negative women can actually be treated. Aspects of healthcare infrastructure include how much of the treatment, qualified healthcare personnel, and the clinics are available. Sticking with the analogy of a ship's expedition, if the objective is the elimination of Rh disease, then the ship itself represents the developing world's infrastructure. Just like how the components of a ship must be sufficient for the journey being undertaken, the level of a nation's infrastructure must be suitably equipped to treat Rh disease. Furthermore, in addition to the integrity of the ship, ample fuel is also required to reach the intended destination.

ECONOMIC QUESTIONS

You might have already guessed that the fuel in this analogy is monetary funding. It is no secret that financial commitments are necessary in order to facilitate infrastructural upgrades. Regarding the economics associated with the elimination of Rh disease, there are a couple of complex questions that arise. There are the obvious ones that arise such as *"how much will it cost the developed world to upgrade their infrastructure to accomplish the goal of Rh disease eradication?"* and *"do nations within the developing world have the economic resources to invest in a project like this?"*. Although these questions are complex, their complexity lies in the intricate evaluation of a nation's resources and the specificity of the case-by-case nature of the questions. Instead, more thought provoking questions would be "what sectors would funds have to be allocated to?" and "how can the developing world accomplish the goal of Rh disease eradication in a cost effective manner?".

A nation's economic profile is described by its activity in each of four economic sectors. Developing countries can usually attribute a larger percentage of their GDP to the primary and secondary economic sectors that are concerned with activities like agriculture and manufacturing respectively (Paprotny, 2021). The economies of developed countries on the other hand have progressed beyond a reliance on industrialization (Paprotny, 2021). Instead, they can attribute a larger portion of their GDP to the tertiary and quaternary sectors of the economy (Paprotny, 2021). The tertiary economic sector is concerned with occupations related to manufactured goods, such as the sale, transportation or exchange of those products (Paprotny, 2021). Finally, the quaternary sector deals with the acquisition of knowledge, these include the subsectors of education and research & development (Paprotny, 2021). In the section above, limiting aspects of healthcare infrastructure, including available quantities of the treatment and available healthcare personnel, were mentioned. These potential shortcomings highlight that an emphasis should be placed on funding for the education and research & development sectors if the developing world wishes to thoroughly eliminate Rh disease (Shiffman & Smith, 2007). It was found that greater investments in the research & development of the healthcare sector correlated with better health outcomes for developing nation populations (Lansang & Dennis, 2004). Hence, if developing countries wish to eradicate Rh disease in the long run, investing in the infrastructure to do so would be beneficial. The specific type of infrastructure required to eradicate Rh disease is addressed in chapter 11.

In order to facilitate those operations, developing countries would require qualified personnel to carry out these R&D projects. It is important to note that the margin of error for these projects are slimmer when being conducted in the developing world, due to their limited budget. To ensure the success of these R&D endeavours, developing nations must employ the best and brightest minds accessible. Hiring experts from beyond the borders of the developing world is an option, however this method would incur greater costs. Investing in the education sub-sector would decrease costs in the long run, by developing homegrown talent, however it would take longer. Due to this longer timeline, more women and babies would suffer needlessly. This leaves decision makers within the developing world in a tough predicament.

POLITICAL QUESTIONS

Speaking of decision makers, they play arguably the most important role in determining whether or not Rh disease is eliminated. In our analogy, decision makers represent the crewmates responsible for the navigation of the ship. From the section above, you can see why. The governing bodies of developing countries have the final say in which sectors receive funding and how much funding is allocated to them. The head of state in a developing country is essentially the captain of the ship. So in order to fully eradicate Rh disease within the borders of developing nations, leaders of these nations would have to make it priority. The issue is that there are numerous problems developing countries have to deal with. These countries experience complications such as environmental disasters, economic turmoil and food shortages (Walt & Gilson, 1994). Developed countries also run into these problems, but because they have more resources available they are not hit as hard as developing countries are. For argument sake, let's imagine that these external threats to human health do not exist. This scenario raises an interesting question, *"if the eradication of Rh disease was the main priority in developing nations, would they be able to achieve this goal?"*.

Based on previous research, it appears that most developing countries would still have some difficulty doing so (Bhutani et al, 2013). Usually when someone finds that cannot accomplish a goal on their own, they will seek out help. Going with this logic, the following question arises:*"if political leaders in the developing world cannot eradicate Rh disease on their own, who should they ask for help?"*. Setting aside the issue of inadequate infrastructure, it appears that developing countries generally do not include the opinion of key stakeholders when creating policies related to healthcare (Walt & Gilson, 1994). Stakeholders are individuals that have some interest in the issue at hand, in this case Rh disease, and getting their input is expected to yield results (Shiffman & Smith, 2007). Stakeholders, such as citizens in areas heavily burdened by Rh disease complications, could provide a unique perspective that government officials cannot (Shiffman & Smith, 2007). In addition to this, these internal stakeholders will continue to advocate on behalf of afflicted individuals, to ensure that the issue is not forgotten about in the future (Shiffman & Smith, 2007). These internal stakeholders can be thought of as ship staff that verify the tickets of the ship's passengers, they make sure everyone is accounted for along the trip to the destination.

Stakeholders from outside affected communities can also provide many benefits to eliminating Rh disease. Global health initiatives, like WIRhE—mentioned in chapter 7—provide numerous benefits. The first is that global health initiatives can help with the lack of funding. Philanthropic activity in the discipline of global health has been increasing over the years (Jung & Harrow, 2019). Reputable NGOs provide legitimacy that philanthropists value when pledging large sums of monetary funds to global health initiatives. In addition to this, these organizations employ valuable experts that have the capability to create road maps to ensure concrete goals are achieved. In the metaphorical sense, these NGOs represent an external navigation team that communicates with the crew on board. In essence, they make sure that the ship stays on its intended course, so that the passengers may eventually reach the intended destination.

SOCIOCULTURAL QUESTIONS

The passengers traveling on this literary device represent the individuals in the developing world that are affected by Rh disease. In this chapter we have been speaking about Rh disease as if it only affects fetuses and newborns, when in reality it devastates entire families. A lack of knowledge, within developing populations on Rh disease is cited to be one explanation for the higher burden experienced by the same population (Pegoraro et al, 2020). It is suggested that educating the citizens of these developing nations on Rh disease, would result in a decrease of Rh-related complications (Pegoraro et al, 2020). This brings up the extremely important question, *"how is Rh education taught in a way that ensures the message gets across effectively?"*. It is important to keep in mind that it is not just a language barrier that must be taken into account, but a cultural one as well.

If Rh educational interventions are conducted in developing countries without considering the sociocultural landscape, it could actually alienate certain members of the population. Women across the globe, from both the developed and developing world, continue to experience unfair treatment due to their gender. In a study conducted in developing countries, mistreatment during childbirth was noted as a fairly common occurrence (Balde et al, 2020). In earlier chapters, it was revealed that in order for Rh disease complications to occur, a Rh-negative mother must be pregnant with a Rh positive baby. In the case that this message were to get misconstrued, it could result in the social devaluation of women with Rh-negative status. This scenario reiterates the importance of having internal stakeholders, that are members of the community, who understand how to effectively communicate scientific information to the intended audience.

The issue of access to healthcare was also cited as a reason for a higher prevalence of Rh disease in the developing world (Pegoraro et al, 2020). Something to consider is *"does every citizen of a developing country have the same access to healthcare?"*. From previous studies done in multiple developing countries it was found that there was a significant difference in the quality of care between those of higher socioeconomic status in comparison to those of a lower socioeconomic status (Houghton, Bascolo & Riego, 2020). If we apply this to the issue of Rh disease, it could mean that only Rh-negative women of higher socioeconomic status receive treatment. This scenario would undoubtedly amplify the socioeconomic gap between rich and poor families in the developing world (Lahelma, 2001). This would be the equivalent of only the first class passengers being allowed to embark on the destination in our metaphor. If part of the population is ignored, then the world cannot claim to be free from Rh disease. These situations can be avoided if there is collaboration between political leaders, community members and NGOs when developing these educational workshops. NGOs can work alongside with community members to ensure the message is effectively communicated with creating social repercussions. By listening to the opinions of NGOs and community leaders, the governments of developing countries can also determine which members of the population are most vulnerable. Political leaders also have the ability to create programs and policies to ensure that Rh disease treatment is available to everyone in the population, including these vulnerable ones.

MORE QUESTIONS

This raises ethical questions like *"how does the developing world address the effects of social stratification in terms of treating Rh disease?"* and *"What sort of policies or laws will have to be put in place to protect the individuals at the lower end of social hierarchies?"*. So you see, when we aim to answer the questions surrounding Rh disease increasingly complex questions begin to arise. Furthermore, each developing country has their own unique political and cultural landscape to consider. Due to this fact, the answers to the previously mentioned questions increase in their nuance when you apply them on a case by case basis. When it comes to Rh disease, it is important to understand that there is no "one size fits all" framework that can be applied.

What we do know is that developing nations will have to work side by side with key stakeholders, like community members and NGOs, to incorporate a multidisciplinary approach in order to fully eradicate Rh disease. It will also require a vigilant effort from project leaders to ensure that new questions are taken note of when they arise. By doing so the world will have a better chance at changing the global estimate from 276 newborns per 100,000 live births affected by Rh disease to zero.

CONCLUSION

To summarize, even though there are effective treatments against Rh disease, it continues to have an impact on the lives of families world-wide. There are many unanswered questions regarding Rh disease, particularly pertaining to the developing world, Unanswered questions about Rh disease regarding infrastructure include determining *"how many individuals are susceptible to the disease?"* and *"what strategies can be used with the current infrastructure to eradicate Rh disease?"*. Economic questions related to the cost of eradicating Rh disease and what sectors require the most funding in order to do so also remain unanswered. In addition to this, those leading the Rh eradication effort must also be carefully chosen. Unique sociocultural factors of each developing country bring about challenges when it comes to the elimination of Rh disease. Because of the multidisciplinary relationship required to eradicate Rh disease, new questions about Rh disease will continue to arise as previous ones receive answers. The next chapter will examine the treatments available for Rh disease as well as their efficiency.

CHAPTER 9

What is the Treatment for RH Disease and How Efficient is It?

*Written By **Salma Abrahim***

I N SPITE OF THE UNCERTAINTY and questions that come with Rh disease, there are many treatment options available. Although 50% of all Rh disease cases will not require any treatment and are considered mild, monitoring the infant's health pre and post-delivery is critical in case serious issues start to develop (NHS, 2018).There are many treatments for Rh disease that are available, depending on the severity and the accessibility of resources. The following types of treatments will be discussed in this chapter: Rh D immunoglobulin, intravenous immunoglobulin, plasma exchange, intrauterine intravascular transfusion, phototherapy and two types of medicinal treatments: colony stimulating factors and competitive heme oxygenase inhibitors. This chapter will have sensitive information regarding maternal-fetal health, and this is a disclaimer regarding these topics.

FETOMATERNAL HEMORRHAGE TESTING

For mothers who are Rh-negative and have been exposed to Rh-positive blood from the fetus, assessing fetomaternal hemorrhage (the entry of fetal blood into the maternal circulation) is critical (Costumbrado et al., 2020). Maternal sensitization occurs when a Rh-negative mother is exposed to a Rh D antigen through carrying a Rh-positive fetus

(Costumbrado et al., 2020). In 75% of pregnant women, transplacental (crossing the placenta) passage of fetal red blood cells occurs, either during delivery or during pregnancy (Ramasethu, 2004). With advancing gestational age (how far along the pregnancy is), or with the prevalence of fetomaternal transfusion (when the mother and fetus undergo blood transfer) there is a 64% chance of transfusion occurring during delivery (Ramasethu, 2004). Following delivery, the volume of fetal blood that is present in maternal circulation of 96% of women is less than 1 ml, but even small amounts of blood are enough to cause sensitization (Ramasethu, 2004). The exact amount of fetal blood that is Rh-positive needed to sensitize the mother varies, but most mothers are sensitized in as small as 0.01 ml of blood (Ramasethu, 2004). Fetomaternal hemorrhage can be assessed via the Rosette test, and the fetal cells appear pink in colour and are considered positive screens. The rosette test begins with the process of incubating maternal Rh-negative blood with anti-Rho (D) immunoglobulin to separate the maternal from the fetal cells (Krywko et al., 2020). The maternal cells are not bonded to the immunoglobulin as they are Rho (D) negative (Krywko et al., 2020). Rho (D) immunoglobulin is an antibody that is made from human plasma and targets the red blood cells in the sample (Urbaniak & Greiss, 2000). Any Rh-positive fetal cells in the maternal blood sample are bound to the immunoglobulin (Krywko et al., 2020). Indicator cells with enzymes are added, and they solely bind to the fetal cells that were sensitized in the sample, and the rosette patterns of the cells can be viewed under a microscope (Krywko et al., 2020).

The screens can be confirmed with a Kleihauer-Betke (KB) test (Costumbrado et al., 2020). The KB test will dictate the percentage or ratio of fetal red blood cells to maternal red blood cells, in addition to fetal blood cells with hemoglobin F present in maternal blood (Ramasethu, 2004). The test exposes maternal blood to an acidic solution, and Hemoglobin F remains intact in said acidic environment, as maternal cells with hemoglobin A (adult hemoglobin) is removed and is denatured (Krywko et al., 2020). Hemoglobin F is the main oxygen carrying protein present in fetal blood, and composes between 60 to 80 percent of total hemoglobin content in a mature newborn, and by targeting hemoglobin F in the test, we are able to identify the quantity of fetal blood in maternal circulation (Steinberg & Thein, 2021). The smear is then stained with a solution, and the fetal blood cells appear pink in color, while maternal cells appear clear (Krywko et al., 2020).

RH D IMMUNOGLOBULIN (RHIG)

One of the main objectives for the management of RH disease is the prevention of maternal sensitization (Costumbrado et al., 2020). If the mother's exposure to the Rh D antigen occurs during her first pregnancy, the fetus is frequently delivered before any anti-D antigens are created and the pregnancy is not typically affected (Costumbrado et al., 2020). If the mother has been sensitized and exposed to the Rh D antigen during her first pregnancy, any future pregnancies are at risk to develop HDN (hemolytic disease of the neonate) and, if the fetus is Rh-positive, Rh incompatibility (Costumbrado et al., 2020). Rh incompatibility refers to the condition that develops when a pregnant woman has Rh-negative blood, and the fetus has Rh-positive blood (Kaneshiro & Zieve, 2019). Rhesus factor is a protein that is found on the outside of red blood cells, and people are either Rh-negative and do not have the protein, or Rh-positive and do have the protein on their cells (Cleveland, 2018). In regards to maternal sensitization, Rh D immunoglobulin (RhIg) is able to make a significant contribution in preventing Rh disease from occuring in the mother. RhIg has anti-Rh D antibodies that target Rh-positive erythrocytes, which are cleared out by the spleen and reduces the chance of having Rh disease (Costumbrado et al., 2020) (Yoham &, Casadesus et al., 2020). RhIg is efficient, and has the ability to reduce the rate of alloimmunization (the immune system's response when exposed to foreign antigens) from 16% to less than 1%, and decrease the prevalence of HDN to less than 1% (Costumbrado et al., 2020) (Mota, 2013).

If the mother is suspected to have Rh incompatibility during pregnancy, RhIg is provided as a treatment at 28 weeks gestation (Costumbrado et al., 2020). After delivery, if the newborn is Rh-positive, the mother is treated with RhIg within 72 hours of delivery to decrease the rate of red blood cell destruction (Costumbrado et al., 2020). Partial protection against maternal sensitization can be achieved if RhIg is administered within 13 to 28 days post delivery- administering RhIg at a delayed rate decreases its protective capacity (Yoham & Casadesus, 2020).

In terms of the frequency of doses, the American College of Obstetricians and Gynecologists (ACOG) recommends that once Rh-negative mothers give birth to Rh-positive neonates, they should undergo qualitative and quantitative assessments to determine correct dosage (Costumbrado et al., 2020). These tests are the rosette assay and KB test- used previously to assess fetomaternal hemorrhage. Common adverse effects include headache, dizziness, hypertension and hyperkinetic (abnormal/involuntary) muscle activity, while more serious effects including severe kidney problems and in some cases, death (Yoham & Casadesus, 2020).

If sensitization has occurred, other treatment options are open, such as: intravenous immunoglobulin, plasma exchange, intrauterine transfusion and direct intravascular transfusion (Urbaniak & Greiss, 2000). With the diverse treatment options, and substantial fetal medicine advancements, affected fetuses with HDN have a survival rate of greater than 90% (Urbaniak & Greiss, 2000).

PLASMA EXCHANGE

Plasma exchange requires the removal of 4-5 liters of plasma from the blood containing anti-D antibodies from the mother, and replacing it with albumin/crystalloid solution, which is a replacement fluid for the plasma (Urbaniak & Greiss, 2000). Removing the anti-D antibodies from the mother reduces the levels of the antibodies in maternal circulation (Urbaniak & Greiss, 2000). Plasma exchange has a debatable efficacy rate, and the process would need to be repeated multiple times a week to preserve the reduced levels of anti-D (Urbaniak & Greiss, 2000). In addition, this procedure is strenuous and should not be a primary treatment choice for the mother (Urbaniak & Greiss, 2000). If there is a history of fetal loss from RH disease or the probability that their father is homozygous for RhD, plasma exchange can be facilitated early in the pregnancy depending on the resources available (Urbaniak & Greiss, 2000).

For fetal treatments, analysis of amniotic fluid will determine critical levels of bilirubin and the needed treatments. The possibility of a premature delivery for HDN is chosen if the fetus is judged to be viable in terms of maturity and size (Urbaniak & Greiss, 2000). If delivery is not a viable option, fetal transfusion can be facilitated, while postnatal therapeutic measures include phototherapy (involves light oxidizing bilirubin to water-soluble molecules that are excreted from the body) (Urbaniak & Greiss, 2000).

INTRAVASCULAR INTRAUTERINE TRANSFUSION

Intravascular intrauterine transfusion is the main method of management for severe alloimmunization during pregnancy, and the method involves providing blood to a fetus who is Rh-positive as the fetal red blood cells are continuously being destroyed by the Rh antibodies (Marshall et al., 2019). This treatment is a temporary option until the fetus is considered healthy and mature enough to be delivered safely (Marshall et al., 2019). The transfusion is commonly administered through the umbilical artery or vein, or through the fetal abdomen (Marshall et al., 2019). Transfusion through the umbilical vessel is the preferred method of delivery as there is a higher survival rate than administration through the fetal abdomen (Marshall et al., 2019). The process involves using an ultrasound to lead the needle into the umbilical vessels or fetal abdomen, while compatible blood type (that is Rh-negative) is supplied and the mother is given antibiotics to prevent infection (Marshall et al., 2019). These transfusions are high risk and may cause preterm labour, fluid leakage from the amniotic sac or fetal death, but the effectiveness of the treatment is high (Marshall et al., 2019). If fetal hydrops is present (a serious condition caused by Rh

WHAT IN THE WORLD IS RH DISEASE?

sensitization), the fetus has 75% chance of survival, and fetuses that do not have hydrops have a 90% chance of survival (Marshall et al., 2019). Transfusion can also be done post-delivery, where some of the infant's blood that has a high level of bilirubin and antibodies can be removed and is replaced with blood from a donor that is suitable for the infant's blood type (NHS, 2018). This process is usually done through an intravenous cannula (using a tube inserted through a vein), and it can additionally add to the infant's current red blood cell count (NHS, 2018).

PHOTOTHERAPY

Phototherapy is a safe treatment option for infants after delivery, and can often reduce the need for a blood transfusion (NHS, 2018). As increased levels of bilirubin in the infant's blood is a sign of Rh incompatibility, phototherapy aids will increase the rate of bilirubin exiting the infant's body (Ernst, 2018). Through a process known as photo-oxidation, the fluorescent light is absorbed by the infant's skin and oxygen is added to the bilirubin in the blood (NHS, 2018). By oxidizing bilirubin, the baby's liver can easily break it down and remove it from the body (NHS, 2018). The treatment involves placing the newborn under fluorescent light, with their eyes protected (NHS, 2018). During the process, intra-venous hydration is administered to the infant as increased levels of water is lost through the baby's skin, and increased levels of urine is being produced (NHS, 2018). The efficacy rate of phototherapy is dependent on size and type of lamp used, in addition to the spectrum of light being delivered (Wagle, 2021). If fluorescent tubes are used, they are placed as close to the infant as possible to maximize irradiance (the power that is received by the infant's body per unit of area)(Wagle, 2021). However, if a halogen light source will be used, the distance to the infant is determined per the instructions set by the manufacturer as this type of light can cause bodily burns (Wagle, 2021). With both types of sources, there is minimal ultraviolet (UV) radiation emitted as the plexiglass covering the tubes absorbs said rays, and the occurrence of erythema (the redness of the skin that is caused by increase blood flow) is not of concern (Wagle, 2021). Temporary side effects might include loose stools and skin rashes (Wong & Bhutani, 2021). The most effective region of the visible light spectrum for this treatment is blue-green (425-490 nm), and for maximum exposure the sides of the infant's bassinet should be lined with aluminium foil or white cloth to increase surface area (Wagle, 2021). An alternative method involves placing the infant on a blanket that contains optical fibers, and lights travel through the fibers to the infant's back- a process known as fiber optic phototherapy (NHS, 2018).

INTRAVENOUS IMMUNOGLOBULIN FOR INFANTS

Alongside phototherapy, treatment with intravenous immunoglobulin (IVIG) can be used if the infant's bilirubin level is continuing to rise (NHS, 2018). This treatment is similar to the RhIG administered to mothers that we discussed in a previous paragraph. The solution is composed of antibodies (proteins that the immune system produces to fight off organisms that carry diseases) taken from healthy donors and injected into the infant's vein (NHS, 2018). When Rh disease occurs, maternal antibodies in the infant's blood attach to the antigen receptors on the infant's red blood cells, and it triggers the destruction of the antigen-antibody complex, while destructing the red blood cell itself at the same time (Ahmed, 2017). The immunoglobulin helps with blocking the antibody-antigen complex receptor, and the antibodies are not able to bind to their receptor- and therefore cannot promote the death of the red blood cells (Ahmed, 2017). This mechanism will also help with decreasing the bilirubin level, reducing the chance of needing an intravascular intrauterine transfusion and decreasing the duration of needed phototherapy sessions for the infant (NHS, 2018) (Ahmed, 2017). There are risks associated with IVIG, such as an allergic reaction from the immunoglobulin but the severity is unknown and can vary (NHS, 2018). Therefore, with the vague side effects, and the restricted supply of IVIG that is present for treatment, this type of therapy is only used if the infant's bilirubin levels are rising at a rapid pace, or during severe cases of Rh disease (where IVIG can be administered during pregnancy) (NHS, 2018).

ORAL DRUGS FOR INFANTS

There are two types of oral drugs that are normally administered to infants with Rh disease, and they can either be colony stimulating factors or competitive heme oxygenase inhibitors (Wagle, 2021). Firstly, colony stimulating factors are composed of glycoproteins that are produced from modified mammalian cells for erythropoietin (EPO) (Dulay, 2020). Erythropoietin is a hormone produced by the kidneys, and it plays a critical role in producing red blood cells and carrying oxygen around the body ("Erythropoietin", 2011). The activity of the drug induced EPO mimics endogenous (naturally originating) EPO, and simulates division of erythroid cells to release reticulocytes (immature red blood cells) in the bloodstream (Dulay, 2020). It can be used to treat anemia, a condition that is a result of the destruction of red blood cells when they are not able to carry needed oxygen to the infant's muscles (Dulay, 2020). Anemia from Rh disease can be diagnosed via a percutaneous (through the skin) umbilical cord blood sampling (Dulay, 2020).

Secondly, competitive heme oxygenase inhibitors are composed of hemoglobin that aid with the blockage of hemoglobin oxygenase (HO-1), which is a rate-limiting enzyme in the production of bilirubin (Wagle, 2021). This process halts the conversion of hemoglobin (because it blocks HO-1) to bilirubin, and the heme is not stored in the tissues and is excreted in the bile (Wagle, 2021). This drug does not interact with the infant's DNA and therefore cannot and therefore it has no effect on bilirubin that has been previously formed in the infant's blood (Wagle, 2021). Previous studies have shown that oxygen inhibitors are effective in blocking and preventing the progression of jaundice levels, and phototherapy was terminated in 97% of infants (Wagle, 2021).

With advancing neonatal medical care and research, there are an array of treatment options available for Rh disease, depending on disease progression and maternal-fetal health. Qualitative and quantitative assessments are administered to determine the best treatment method and, as alluded to earlier, the prevention of maternal sensitization is the main objective of care with Rh disease. Treatment options include immunoglobulin, plasma exchange, blood transfusion, phototherapy and medicinal treatments. The next chapter will explain how Rh disease is discussed in popular media, and potential conspiracy theories surrounding it.

CHAPTER 10

How is RH Disease Talked about in Society?

Written By **Joonsoo Sean Lyeo, Rahma Gulaid,**
& **Olivia Brodowski**

INTRODUCTION

The following chapter provides some insight into various popular media and journal articles which examine the lesser known and even contentious, perspectives regarding Rh Disease. Some of the topics discussed in this chapter include conspiracy theories around Rh disease, the ethical implications of contemporary treatments for Rh disease, and alternative treatments for Rh disease. These topics have been explored by multiple contributors, who sought to summarize some of the broader and more unique perspectives surrounding discussions of Rh disease.

HOW HAS RH DISEASE BEEN DISCUSSED IN POPULAR MEDIA?

In cases where an Rh-positive fetus' red blood cells are being destroyed by the Rh-sensitized mother's immune system, an intrauterine transfusion can save the fetus' life. Such severe cases are easily avoidable by administering immunoprophylaxis during pregnancy. However, any preventative measures are up to the discretion of the patient, having full freedom to refuse any Rh(D) treatment. Jehovah's witnesses often reject blood transfusions because they believe the Bible strongly asserts against the storage and consumption of blood. This conflict between physician paternalism— the strong moral will to save lives— and religious ethical beliefs has put lives at risk, including the lives of fetuses. Increasingly, "fewer infants require exchange transfusion for haemolytic disease of the newborn when a high dose of intravenous immunoglobulin is used" (Lakatos, 2004, p. 1076). Medical practices which are sensitive to the ethical considerations and restrictions of religious patients, such as Jehovah's Witnesses, are becoming more and more commonplace. In this case, "'bloodless' solutions" (1076) forthe treatment of Rh disease are becoming more available and more efficacious.

One of these 'bloodless' solutions was demonstrated in a case in 1999 where "an AB0 incompatible term infant girl [was] born to parents who were Jehovah's Witnesses" (1076). Instead of receiving blood transfusions, alternative treatments included oral admission of D-pen-icillamine, phototherapy, intravenous fluids, and recombinant human erythropoietin.These treatments are discussed in more detail in the previous chapter. In the end, the infant's "physical growth and motor milestones at 3 years of age revealed no red flags for neurodevelop-mental maturation" (1076).

A key takeaway from this example is that by pushing physicians to find alternative treatments, when such treatments are successful, they can be employed more broadly, making them more accessible to everyone. D-penicillamine treatments in combination with phototherapy seem to diminish the intensity of hyperbilirubinemia, a debilitating consequence of HDN. On top of this, D-penicillamine "is able to prevent the possible adverse side effects of phototherapy that have been shown in vitro and most recently in vivo" (1076). What started off as an incongruity between religious ethics and medical care has resulted in finding innovative ways to treat patients with specific considerations. Such innovative treatments help the medical community on a grander scale simply by making treatment more available to everyone.

HOW IS RH DISEASE DISCUSSED AROUND THE WORLD?

As mentioned, treatment of RH disease is at the discretion of the patient, hence one of the primary methods of rhesus prevention is awareness. These advocacy and education campaigns are conducted differently all across the world.

According to a study conducted in Enugu, Nigeria, 4.5%. out of 6306 women were Rh D negative. (Okeke, Ocheni, Nwagha, & Ibegbulam, 2011) Several informational campaigns have been launched in Nigeria as methods of loss prevention. The Rhesus Solution Initiative, a non-profit that aims to create an awareness of rhesus incompatibility, is one such example. The organization advocates for Rh negative women in Lagos and Nigeria, by fighting for the safe monitoring of at-risk pregnancy and the availability of blood testing, and the providing of immediate blood donations. They promote awareness of the disease primarily to women in rural areas that would otherwise not have access to treatment and information. (Rhesus Solution Initiative) Moreover, they have provided postpartum rhesus prophylaxis to more than 10 000 women. (Zipursky, Bhutani, & Odame, 2018)

A study conducted in Bisha, Saudia Arabia found that of 108 participants, 11.1% presented a negative blood group. Researchers concluded that these results were comparative to other populations. However, they argued that the mere 41.5% of women aware of the risks of RH-negative pregnancy was substandard. The study also noted the association between awareness, age and education. Older women and uneducated women are at a higher risk due to a lack of information, hence investigators concluded that educational programs had to be introduced to address this gap. (Yahia, Miskeen, Sohail, Algak, & Aljadran, 2020)

The issue present in Brazil differs from Nigeria and Saudi Arabia, because it is one of infrastructure as opposed to public discourse, however the results are just as detrimental. A survey was conducted on a multitude of Brazilian healthcare workers to provide both national and regional reporting on RH sensitization. The study revealed large knowledge gaps amongst the medical professionals. They struggled to answer basic questions such as what type of Rh immunoglobulin is used in treatment, and at what point in the pregnancy the mother receives it. They also struggled to determine whether their institutions had Rh screenings or the cost of the immunoglobulin. These lapses in judgement may greatly affect a patient's treatment. A higher level of attention would be a beneficial step in disease prevention. (Varianea & Sant'Annab, 2020). This in turn contributes to the continued risk of RH disease. As such, a central aim in global prevention must be the promotion of educational campaigns.

Although many high income countries have almost eradicated the illness, a lack of prevalence can result in a lack of awareness. Low public awareness fosters the spread of misinformation, which may result in hesitation to have treatment. An example of how a decreased understanding can manifest into a public health crisis is the spike in parental refusal of essential vaccines. In 2017, 28.4% of American children 19 to 35 months old had not received their seven-part measles vaccination. (Hortez, 2017) As a result we have seen outbreaks of preventable disease, such as measles. In 2019, the United States confirmed 1,282 individual cases of measles. A dramatic increase from the mere 55 cases reported in 2012. (Centers for Disease Control and Prevention) Moreover, a lack of medical understanding creates a breeding ground for conspiracy theories.

ARE THERE ANY CONSPIRACY THEORIES SURROUNDING RH DISEASE?

A deeper dive into the non-academic discourse around Rh disease, and around Rh blood types in general, reveals a bizarre web of conspiracy theories and dubious pseudoscience embraced by online fringe communities. Before proceeding, it should be acknowledged that the following conspiracy theories are not substantiated by credible academic evidence. For instance, some of these online fringe communities claim that Rh disease is the result of the mother and the child being different species

(Zad, Khobragade & Saache, 2018). Similar ideas have been espoused by the self-proclaimed 'cryptozoologist and ufologist' Nick Redfern, who argues that individuals with Rh negative blood are the product of "extraterrestrials manipulating the human bloodline in the distant past" (Redfern, 2015). In support of his argument, Redfern claims that individuals with Rh negative blood are more likely to be interested in UFOs, possess stronger psychic abilities, and typically have a higher IQ (Redfern, 2015). It should be noted that Redfern provides no evidence to substantiate these claims. Redfern also claims that individuals with Rh negative blood are "resilient to illness, virus, and disease"; however there is substantial evidence to suggest that the opposite is true, and that individuals with Rh negative blood are actually more susceptible to worse health outcomes and health disorders (Flegr, Hoffmann, & Dammann, 2015).

Other online fringe communities allege that Rh disease is the result of cross-breeding between humans and a race of reptilian beings (Adams, 2016). To this end, they often claim that the high prevalence of miscarriages and stillbirths among Rh negative mothers is the result of some sort of inherent genetic incompatibility with their offspring (Zad, Khobragade & Saache, 2018). Some members of these online fringe communities even claim that those with Rh negative blood share 'reptilian' physical characteristics, for example lower-than-average body temperatures and extra vertebrae (Adams, 2016). It should be noted that, within academic circles, there is currently no credible evidence to support the association between Rh negative blood and body temperature; and while an estimated 7% to 30% of people have an extra vertebrae in their lower spine region, there is also no evidence to suggest that this anomaly is associated with the prevalence of Rh negative blood (Sekharappa, Amritanand & Venkatesh Krishnan, 2014).

Other online fringe communities suggest that the higher prevalence of Rh negative blood types in certain ethnic groups is somehow indicative of the superiority of these groups (Adams, 2016). These sentiments have been espoused by a small subset of the Basque community, who point out that approximately 20% to 40% of ethnic Basques possess Rh negative blood (Khan, 2020). This has led some Basquophiles to claim that modern Basques are the 'purest' descendants of the Cro-Magnons, the first of the modern humans to settle in Europe (Khan, 2020). This notion has largely been debunked, as several genetic studies indicate that modern Basques are no more representative of the ancestral gene pool than other European ethnicities (Alonso et al., 2005). These findings have not deterred Santiago Sevilla, a self-proclaimed historian of Basque heritage, from assigning them a near-mystical quality. In his books, Sevilla claims that the Basques were the true builders of Stonehenge and had settled the Americas long before the Age of Exploration (Sevilla, 2018).

ARE THERE ANY POPULAR ALTERNATIVE TREATMENTS FOR RH DISEASE?

In many parts of the world, different cultures have developed their own traditional remedies for the treatment of Rh disease. There is only limited evidence for the efficacy and safety of many of the remedies discussed in this section, which should be taken into account when reading the following text. That being said, while they may not receive support from the realm of evidence based medicine, the traditional remedies discussed below do provide interesting insight into the conservation of traditional knowledge and practices.

For instance, the Igbo people of Nigeria have developed several unique, ethnocultural traditions and healing rituals dedicated to curing families of serial miscarriages and repeated infant deaths (Ilechukwu, 2007). It is now known that a significant portion of these perinatal deaths are the result of Rh incompatibility. That being said, it should be noted that in many Igbo communities these deaths have historically been, and continue to be, attributed to ogbanje; a term referring to souls that are believed to be stuck in a rapidly alternating cycle between life and death (Umoh & Akinola, 1994). As local traditions state, ogbanje are destined to be repeatedly born to the same mother until this cycle is broken. Some Igbo healing rituals aim to cure serial miscarriages by freeing these souls (Umoh & Akinola, 1994). For instance, there are accounts of faith healers prescribing holy water, through divinations and rituals, to guide expectant mothers through their pregnancies and ensure the safety of their children (Holter, 2014). Expectant mothers may also meet with their families to pray for the health and survival of their children during pregnancy and birth (Ilechukwu, 2007). As a result, prayer houses and faith healers are often favoured over hospitals, especially in rural communities. This lack of proper medical treatment contributes to increased perinatal death rates (Umoh & Akinola, 1994).

Popular alternative treatments for Rh disease can also be found in other cultures. For instance, there are several traditional Chinese medicines and remedies that are often administered in the treatment of recurrent miscarriages caused by Rh incompatibility (Bian et al., 1998). One herbal remedy which enjoys a fair amount of popularity is the Yi Guan Jian decoction, created from the boiling and distilling of six types of medicinal herbs (Hullender Rubin, Cantor & Marx, 2013). The herbs in this concoction are chosen for their supposed ability to circulate Qi, a vital energy, and nourish Yin, a passive energy (Hullender Rubin, Cantor & Marx, 2013). Other forms of traditional healing, such as acupuncture and foot baths, may also be administered alongside these herbal remedies (Hullender Rubin, Cantor & Marx, 2013). While there is some limited evidence to support the safety and effectiveness of these remedies, the quality of studies putting forward these claims are generally poor and warrant further investigation (Li et al., 2016).

Herbal remedies for Rh disease can also be found in many other cultures. For instance, in the ethnic Oromian communities of Ethiopia, many traditional healers consider the ground shrub *Sida schimperiana* to be an effective herbal remedy for the treatment of *shotelaye*, a local term for Rh disease (Tesfaye et al., 2020). The alleged healing properties of this herb have also been recognized by Ethiopian Orthodox monks at the Debre Libanos monastery, who recommend a healing ritual in which a portion of the herb is tied around the waist or forehead of the affected mother (Teklehaymanot et al., 2007). Elsewhere in Ethiopia, traditional healers recommend the use of a different medicinal herb, *Achyranthes aspera*, in the treatment of Rh disease (Kefalew, Asfaw & Kelbessa, 2015). As part of a healing ritual, traditional healers cut the roots of this herb into small parts while issuing a prayer (Kefalew, Asfaw & Kelbessa, 2015). The roots are then combined with brown teff, black malt, and buckthorn to form a liquid concoction, which is then provided to patients to drink over the course of the next three days (Kefalew, Asfaw & Kelbessa, 2015).

Similar practices can be seen among traditional healers in Qatar, who recommend the use of certain herbal remedies to 'cleanse' a woman's uterus after a miscarriage caused by Rh disease (Kilshaw et al., 2016). Conversely, due to the popularity of herbal medicine in the Middle East, some traditional healers recommend against the use of certain herbs during pregnancy because of their perceived effects on uterine function (Kilshaw et al., 2016). Examples of herbs purported to cause miscarriages, as identified by traditional healers, include: red seed, black seed, thyme, helba, sage, cinnamon, and ginger (Kilshaw et al., 2016). To this end, many traditional healers also recommended against the consumption of caffeine and junk food, which they believe put expectant mothers at greater risk of miscarriage (Kilshaw et al., 2017).

This section provides insight into some of the traditional treatments of Rh disease which have been developed by several different ethnocultural communities around the world. Traditional treatments continue to play an important role in the healthcare responses of these communities, especially among groups which lack ready access to modernized healthcare systems (Lezotre, 2014). Before concluding, it should again be acknowledged that compared to evidence-based medicine, in which the safety and effectiveness of medical treatments are validated using the scientific method, there is less evidence to support traditional treatments for Rh disease. That being said, it should be acknowledged that the science around Rh disease is continuing to grow, as will be discussed in the following "Chapter 11: Where is Rh disease research headed in the future?".

CHAPTER 11

Where is RH Disease Research Headed in the Future?

Written By Olivia Brodowski

INTRODUCTION

Within the past two decades, the Rhesus disease has been largely mitigated in the United States and countries in Western Europe. Research from Columbia Irving Medical Center reveals, however, that poorer countries have yet to establish consistent rehabilitation and precautionary practices against the easily preventable Rh disease and neonatal mortality. Columbia Irving's research highlights the crucial factor that: although preventative measures against Rh(D) sensitization— and thus, against Rh disease— was discovered more than fifty years ago, research shows that, worldwide efforts to prevent Rh disease remain below the minimum threshold and far below the optimum goal (Pegoraro et al., 2020, p. 7). This chapter will investigate the potential reasons for the mismanaging of preventative measures against Rh disease as well as implementation measures to counter such mismanaging.

DISCUSSION

Columbia Irving researchers identify that while no countries have maintained acceptable levels of immunoprophylaxis, "regions with the highest gap in absolute numbers are Asia South and Sub-Saharan Africa" (Pegoraro et al., 2020, p. 7). Immunoprophylaxis is the prevention of disease by the production of active or passive immunity through antenatal, the time during pregnancy, and postpartum, the time immediately after childbirth, dose admissions.

An analysis done by the Cochrane Collaboration explains that IgG anti Rh(D) immunoprophylaxis "is recommended for RhD-negative mothers at 28 or 30 weeks of pregnancy and within 72 hours of potential maternal exposure to fetal red cells to prevent the mother developing antibodies during the pregnancy. RhD negative mothers also receive postpartum anti-D after a RhD-positive baby to reduce the risk of sensitization during the next pregnancy" (*Intramuscular versus Intravenous Anti-D for Preventing Rhesus Alloimmunization during Pregnancy,* n.d., p. 2).

Asia South and Sub-Saharan Africa are also "the two regions with the highest incidence of neonatal death due to kernicterus," a rare form of brain damage linked with neonatal jaundice which is often a result of Rh disease. The reasons for the continuing mismanagement of providing both antenatal and postpartum immunoprophylaxis are widely varied; and so, a one-size-fits-all solution does not exist. The reasons range from non-routine Rh blood group typing, high costs of IgG anti-Rh(D) due to privatization, insufficient or unavailability of supplies due to economic or political factors, or simply the neglect of performing immunoprophylaxis despite available resources.

A common angle that researchers and doctors propose in accordance to solving the problem of the continuing existence of Rh disease is increased understanding and awareness of antenatal and postpartum precautions. However, Rh disease has been understood for the last several decades. Research, understanding, and awareness is no longer sufficient. What are some more concrete and proactive measures that can be implemented that are region specific?

Firstly, more accurate data collection regarding the annual amount of IgG anti-Rh(D) doses available within a country compared to the amount of doses actually administered is integral in identifying the initial point of mismanagement. Many countries and regions do not update statistics regarding their administration of IgG anti-Rh(D) which creates a roadblock in identifying the potential root causes of mismanagament. The approximate statistics that are available are a good touchstone for regional and world health organizations to spotlight regions of need; however, that spotlight has already been shone. Proactive next steps are required.

The current spotlight shows that regions across the globe are consistently missing their minimum threshold of IgG anti-Rh(D) dose admissions (Fig 1). However, while still not making their optimum threshold, High Income countries are well above their minimum threshold, revealing a fundamental discrepancy between dose admissions and the economic wellbeing of a country. The minimum threshold describes the admission of postpartum immunoprophylaxis doses *only*. The optimum threshold describes the point where *no* cases of Rh(D) are recorded due to the combination of antenatal *and* postpartum immunoprophylaxis admissions. While this may seem unattainable and unrealistic, the appropriate resources and measures do exist— they just are not being used and enacted to their fullest potential. Columbia Irving distinguishes their regions based on Global Burden of Disease (GBD), Gross Domestic Product (GDP), as well as geographical location. Of the thirty-five countries within the High Income typography, the United States, Norway, and Ireland are the only three *without* government instated public health care policies. Of the Asia South group two out of the six countries: Pakistan and Bhutan, have government health care policies; of the forty-seven countries within the Sub-Saharian Africa group, only nine of them *have* government health care policies. The Asia South and Sub-Saharian Africa group reveal the largest gap between administered IgG anti-Rh(D) dose and the minimum threshold of required doses.

While the correlation is imperfect, the wide gap between administered doses and the minimum threshold coincides with the lack of government instated health care policies, meaning that, simply, the *availability and*

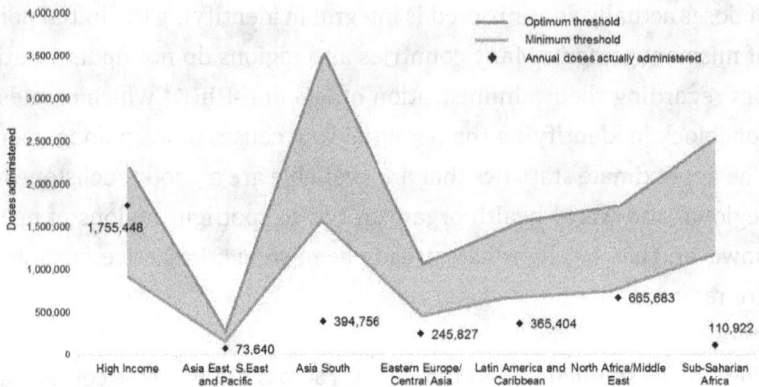

Fig 1. (Pegoraro et al., 2020, p. 5)

accessibility of receiving antenatal and postpartum treatments is lacking in the regions with the largest gaps because their governments are not aiding in that availability and accessibility. Privatized healthcare institutions are sweeping the problem of Rh disease under the rug. A combination of low GDP and privatized health care systems results in the mismanagement of proper IgG anti-Rh(D) admission.

The problem of the persistence of Rh disease is not a simple one. Further research regarding the complexity of this systemic problem would narrow down on the *efficacy of privatized health care systems* in groups with large IgG Rh(D) immunoprophylaxis admission gaps such as Asia South and Sub-Saharian Africa to reveal the potential reason of neglect within prenatal and postpartum care sectors. Data regarding antenatal care and postpartum measures is not readily available and making this adjustment would help specify the area of focus regarding rectifying the problem. However, again, research and data no longer constitute the level of proactivity that is needed. Rather, research and data reveal doors towards the proactivity we are aiming for. What might those doors be?

While it is paramount for future research to identify and mitigate the root cause of the mismanagement of Rh disease preventative measures, it is equally paramount to research and establish foolproof rehabilitative measures before the root problem can be totally eradicated. In other words, affordable, accessible, and long-lasting technology to help fight against severe cases of neonatal jaundice, anemia, and kernicterus— for example— is vital for the time being when grand systemic issues are being questioned.

Researchers identify three main technologies that are regarded as central for reducing severe neonatal health complications and mortality. A universal Visual Assessment of Jaundice, Bilirubin testing, and G-6-PD screening are the three technologies outlined (Slusher et al., 2011).These three technologies and their future implications will be discussed in further detail in the following paragraphs.

UNIVERSAL VISUAL ASSESSMENT OF JAUNDICE

The routine visual monitoring of the onset and progression of Jaundice involves applying pressure on the forehead, mid-sternum, the knee, or ankle to reveal the colour of the underlying skin and tissue. Visual assessments are performed postpartum and throughout the first few weeks after birth. Visual assessment diagrams are the most accessible technology; however, they are also the most likely to produce inaccurate results. Visual easements must be paired with other forms of assessment.

Researchers provide the following standard Visual assessment which is commonly known as the Kramer's Scale (Fig. 2). Close variations of this assessment are commonly used globally. However, the assessment is overall rudimentary and is up to the discretion of the medical advisor which may present inconsistencies. Future research would expand upon currently existing visual assessments to make them more detailed, reducing the instances of discrepancies within results.

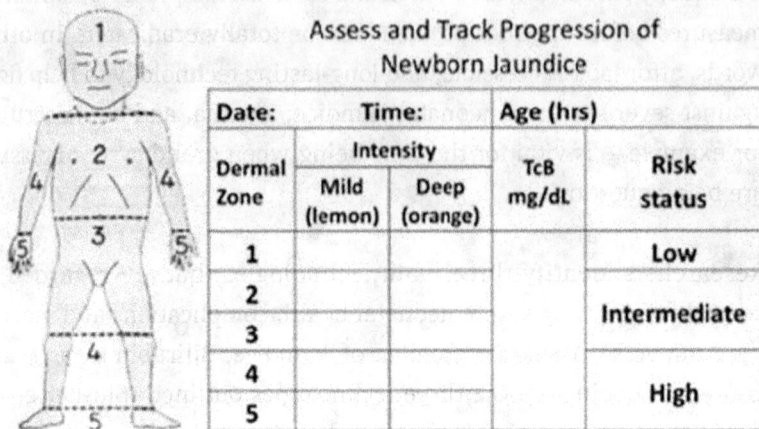

Assess and Track Progression of Newborn Jaundice				
Date:	**Time:**		**Age (hrs)**	
Dermal Zone	**Intensity**		**TcB mg/dL**	**Risk status**
	Mild (lemon)	**Deep (orange)**		
1				Low
2				Intermediate
3				
4				High
5				

Fig. 2 (Rai et al., 2015).

BILIRUBIN TESTING

The Expert American Association of Pediatrics Panel recommends universal bilirubin testing prior to an infant being discharged from the hospital (Slusher et al., 2011, p.187). Infants who had total serum bilirubin measurements as well as transcutaneous bilirubin measurements taken prior to discharge had "better diagnostic ability to predict clinically significant hyperbilirubinemia" (p. 187), meaning that the potential progression of hyperbilirubinemia is easily preventable. This seems like an obvious solution: if an infant's bilirubin levels are tested before discharge, then anomalous cases are more likely to be found, and thus, rectified. So why is testing not standardized?

The same Panel identified that the only current clinical bilirubin screening that is available is an hour-specific nomogram, a diagram which represents the relationship between various parts in a system— such as the different components within the blood. While researchers agree that bilirubin screening is an effective way to detect the potential of hyperbilirubinemia, transcutaneous bilirubin testing may be unreliable during phototherapy because of sunlight's bleaching effect on the skin, device manufacturing inconsistencies, as well as varying measuring results between lighter and darker skin tones. Moreover, the discrepancy of judgement, experience, and expertise between clinicians may result in excessive total serum bilirubin screening which is a painful procedure, exposing newborns to the potential of infection and other related complications. Additionally, researchers highlight that total serum bilirubin screening is costly and time consuming which results in "unnecessary delays in commencing phototherapy and discharge from hospital" (Hussain et al., 2017, p. 1).

Researchers propose that the transcutaneous bilirubinometer (TcBR) is a screening tool used in postnatal wards which has the great potential for near perfect accuracy and time-sensitivity with regards to bilirubin measurement. Transcutaneous bilirubin measurement "devices use multiwavelength spectral reflectance from the skin surface and can be used to estimate total serum or plasma bilirubin and thus avoid blood sampling" (Hussain et al., 2017, p. 1). Transcutaneous bilirubinometers are also point-of-care devices which can be administered as a bed-side test by all levels of healthcare providers including physicians, nurses, and assistants.

Research shows "no significant difference" (Alsaedi, 2018, p. 5) between transcutaneous bilirubin measurements and the more commonly used total serum bilirubin measurement, thus, concluding that TcBR is "accurate and can be performed to monitor bilirubin levels… [leading] to a decrease in the frequency of painful blood sampling" (Alsaedi, 2018, p. 5). Despite this, however, researchers still acknowledge that in cases of severe neonatal jaundice, total serum bilirubin testing, currently, is still the safest form of measurement due to its long history of use by healthcare providers. Future research would expand on current TcBR testing in order to solidify its efficacy and reassure its accuracy among healthcare providers and parents.

G-6-PD SCREENING

G-6-PD deficiency is a genetic disorder wherein the body does not have enough of the enzyme: glucose-6-phosphate dehydrogenase which promotes healthy red blood cells as well as protection from foreign, harmful substances in the blood. Due to its genetic condition, it is most commonly found in males. Researchers state that G-6-PD "is a major contributing cause to neonatal hyperbilirubinemia… [and] a major etiologic factor for kernicterus" (Slusher et al., 2011, p.7). G-6-PD screening is not routinely performed to newborns despite its linkage to severe neonatal health complications.

In 1989 the World Health Organization published comprehensive preventative recommendations regarding the dangerous correlation between G-6-PD and hyperbilirubinemia within neonates. Researchers also highlight, however, that "[d]espite these authoritative recommendations, screening programs have not been adopted universally" (Kaplan et al., 2015, p. 780). The reason for this non implementation is potentially a result of financial and institutional constraints, again, pointing to the privatization of healthcare systems as a central limiting factor of accessible healthcare technologies.

Currently, the mere non-association between G-6-PD and fatal hyperbilirubinemia in newborns is one reason why hyperbilirubinemia can develop. Current research advises parents to take a leading role in limiting exposure of hemolytic agents— substances that are toxic to the blood such as arsenic. Research and practice regarding non painful or intrusive G-6-PD screening measures is lacking and should be taken into consideration for future research.

PROACTIVE NEXT STEPS

It's easy to say that the previously mentioned technologies and screening measures need to be made more affordable for healthcare providers so that they can all be used concurrently. However, how exactly can manufacturers supply such widespread affordability? How can manufacturers be incentivized to produce devices at a lower cost. Who is responsible for initiating those incentives? Meaningful incentives are pivotal in ensuring innovative and competitive product results. The following paragraphs will explore such questions.

Currently, the cost of medical devices in comparison to other health technologies, such as pharmaceuticals, is extremely low primarily because "there is no legal requirement to conduct adequately controlled clinical studies, other than for 'high-risk' devices in some jurisdictions" (Drummond et al., 2016, p. 1055). In the United States, for example, medical devices that are deemed 'low-risk' are only required to demonstrate "reasonable assurance of safety and effectiveness" (Drummond et al., 2016, p. 1055), which substantially cuts down the cost of pricey clinical trials as well as the wait-times for making these devices available for use by healthcare providers. It may seem ill-trustworthy for medical devices to be used in healthcare institutions prior to proper trial, especially in the case where newborns are involved; however, researchers support the efficacy of post-market trials. They assert not to completely outlaw post-market trials because "the performance of the device often depends on the interaction with the user" (Drummond et al., 2016, p. 1055).

For example, conducting post-market trials of transcutaneous bilirubin measurement alongside the more well understood total serum bilirubin measurement, the effectiveness of the transcutaneous bilirubin measurement can be determined post-market with no additional pre-market trial costs, resulting in more affordable accessibility for all regions. In this case, however, a detailed and comprehensive post-market trial guideline must be rigorously followed in order to obtain the most accurate and safe results. To this, further research and next steps may involve outlining and conducting post-market trials on 'low-risk' medical devices such as the transcutaneous bilirubin measurement alongside the more popular and available total serum bilirubin measurement.

By strengthening post-market trial arrangements, testing and research regarding devices can be ongoing, producing more evidence and data than possible in pre-market trials. While medical device registries do currently exist, many of them need improvement with regards to detail, specificity, and comprehensiveness. Such registries would enable all levels of healthcare workers to provide information and feedback regarding 'low-risk' medical devices that otherwise do not receive such attention. Researchers state that such registries "will greatly facilitate the traceability of medical devices and help monitor safety and effectiveness" (Drummond et al., 2016, p. 1057). Additionally, researchers outline various features and functions that such registries should be equipped with. Registries should hold data on multiple devices, should undergo routine updates, and should also include data on the overall treatment patterns of the patient that the device is being used on to monitor timeliness, effectiveness, satisfaction and confidence by the patient.

Post-market clinical trials on 'low risk' medical devices may incentivize device manufactures to keep the cost of their product low and thus, more globally accessible, because rather than a single manufacturer carrying the entire burden of undertaking pre-market clinical trials, the *burden* is spread out between healthcare institutions across the world, seemingly illuminating the *burden* altogether.

CONCLUSION

Rh disease persists today despite the potential of its near eradication. Preventative and rehabilitative measures that are proven to be successful *are out there*, yet neonatal fatality as a result of Rh disease is ongoing. Data shows that regions with higher amounts of privatized healthcare systems also demonstrate higher amounts of cases of Rh disease, and subsequently, neonatal fatality. This demonstrates that the problem of Rh disease is not a simple one; rather, it is a global, systemic one. Further research regarding privatized healthcare systems effectiveness of preventing Rh disease is required. Although, quantitative and qualitative data collection is no longer sufficient. Paired with such further research, the production and incentivization of affordable preventative technologies are a necessary step forward.

REFERENCES

CHAPTER 1

Balick, M. J., & Cox, P. A. (1996). *Plants, people, and culture: the science of ethnobotany.* Scientific American Library.

Barstow, A. L. (1988). On studying witchcraft as women's history: A historiography of the European witch persecutions. *Journal of Feminist Studies in Religion*, 4(2), 7-19.

Baskett, T. F. (2019). From Tragedy to Triumph: Canadian Connections in the Management of Rhesus Hemolytic Disease of the Newborn. *Journal of obstetrics and gynaecology Canada: JOGC= Journal d'obstetrique et gynecologie du Canada: JOGC*, 41, S207-S214.

Bowman, J. (2006). Rh-immunoglobulin: Rh prophylaxis. *Best practice & research. Clinical haematology*, 19(1), 27-34.

Chibi, A. A. (1994). The interpretation and use of divine and natural law in the first marriage crisis of Henry VIII. *Archiv für Reformationsgeschichte*, 85(jg), 265-286.

Clarke, C. A. (1967). Prevention of Rh-haemolytic disease. In *Rhesus haemolytic disease* (pp. 267-269). Springer, Dordrecht.

Costumbrado, J., Mansour, T., & Ghassemzadeh, S. (2020). Rh incompatibility. *StatPearls [Internet]*.

Flores-Bello, A., Mas-Ponte, D., Rosu, M. E., Bosch, E., Calafell, F., & Comas, D. (2018). Sequence diversity of the Rh blood group system in Basques. *European Journal of Human Genetics*, 26(12), 1859-1866.

Golassa, L., Tsegaye, A., Erko, B., & Mamo, H. (2017). High rhesus (Rh (D)) negative frequency and ethnic-group based ABO blood group distribution in Ethiopia. *BMC research notes*, 10(1), 1-5.

Kilshaw, S., Omar, N., Major, S., Mohsen, M., El Taher, F., Al Tamimi, H., ... & Miller, D. (2017). Causal explanations of miscarriage amongst Qataris. BMC Pregnancy and Childbirth, 17(1), 1-12.

Kimball, A. (2019). *The Seed: Infertility is a Feminist Issue.* Coach House Books.

Jackson, M. E., & Baker, J. M. (2021). Hemolytic Disease of the Fetus and Newborn: Historical and Current State. *Clinics in Laboratory Medicine*, 41(1), 133-151.

Levine, P., & Stetson, R. E. (1939). An unusual case of intra-group agglutination. *Journal of the American Medical Association*, 113(2), 126-127.

Liumbruno, G. M., D'Alessandro, A., Rea, F., Piccinini, V., Catalano, L., Calizzani, G., ... & Grazzini, G. (2010). The role of antenatal immunoprophylaxis in the prevention of maternal-foetal anti-Rh (D) alloimmunisation. *Blood transfusion*, 8(1), 8.

Lundevaller, E. H., & Edvinsson, S. (2012). The effect of Rh-negative disease on perinatal mortality: Some evidence from the Skellefteå region, Sweden, 1860–1900. *Biodemography and social biology*, 58(2), 116-132.

Osaro, E., & Charles, A. T. (2010). Rh isoimmunization in Sub-Saharan Africa indicates need for universal access to anti-rhD immunoglobulin and effective management of D-negative pregnancies. *International journal of women's health*, 2, 429.

Queenan, J. T. (2002). Rh-disease: a perinatal success story. *Obstetrics & Gynecology*, 100(3), 405-406.

Rojas, R. E. (2016). *Bad Christians and Hanging Toads* (Doctoral dissertation, Duke University).

Rosse, W. F. (1990). *Clinical immunohematology: basic concepts and clinical applications*. Blackwell Scientific.

Rothenberg, C. E. (2011). Islam on the Internet: the jinn and the objectification of Islam. *The Journal of Religion and Popular Culture*, 23(3), 358-371.

Sisay, M. M., Yirgu, R., Gobezayehu, A. G., & Sibley, L. M. (2014). A qualitative study of attitudes and values surrounding stillbirth and neonatal mortality among grandmothers, mothers, and unmarried girls in rural Amhara and Oromiya regions, Ethiopia: unheard souls in the backyard. *Journal of midwifery & women's health*, 59(s1), S110-S117.

Smith, J. (2000). Regionalism in a New Europe: The Cases of the Basque and Catalan in Spain.

Stockman Iii, J. A. (2001). Overview of the state of the art of Rh disease: history, current clinical management, and recent progress. Journal of pediatric hematology/Oncology, 23(8), 554-562.

Taylor, F. M. (1971). Thomas Linacre: Humanist, Physician, Priest. *The Linacre Quarterly*, 38(3), 17.

Teklehaymanot, T., Giday, M., Medhin, G., & Mekonnen, Y. (2007). Knowledge and use of medicinal plants by people around Debre Libanos monastery in Ethiopia. *Journal of Ethnopharmacology*, 111(2), 271-283.

Touinssi, M., Chiaroni, J., Degioanni, A., De Micco, P., Dutour, O., & Bauduer, F. (2004). Distribution of rhesus blood group system in the French basques: a reappraisal using the allele-specific primers PCR method. *Human heredity*, 58(2), 69-72.

Visser, G. H., Di Renzo, G. C., Spitalnik, S. L., Ayres-de-Campos, D., Escobar, M. F., Barnea, E., ... & Stones, W. (2019). The continuing burden of Rh disease 50 years after the introduction of anti-Rh (D) immunoglobin prophylaxis: call to action. *American journal of obstetrics and gynecology*, 221(3), 227-e1.

Whitley, C. B., & Kramer, K. (2010). A new explanation for the reproductive woes and midlife decline of Henry VIII. *Historical journal*, 827-848.

Whittle, M. J. (1992). Rhesus haemolytic disease. *Archives of disease in childhood*, 67(1 Spec No), 65.

CHATPTER 2

Baskett, T. F. (2019). From Tragedy to Triumph: Canadian Connections in the Management of Rhesus Hemolytic Disease of the Newborn. *Journal of Obstetrics and Gynaecology Canada*, 41, S207–S214. https://doi.org/10.1016/j.jogc.2019.08.038

Darrow, R. R. (1938). *Icterus Gravis (Erythroblastosis) Neonatorum*. https://doi.org/10.1007/978-94-011-6138-1_1

Landsteiner, K., & Wiener, A. S. (1940). An Agglutinable Factor in Human Blood Recognized by Immune Sera for Rhesus Blood. *Proceedings of the Society for Experimental Biology and Medicine*, 43(1), 223–223. https://doi.org/10.3181/00379727-43-11151

Levine, P. (1984). The Discovery of Rh Hemolytic Disease. *Vox Sanguinis*, 47(2), 187–190. https://doi.org/10.1111/j.1423-0410.1984.tb01581.x

Levine, P., Burnham, L., Katzin, E. M., & Vogel, P. (1941). The role of iso-immunization in the pathogenesis of erythroblastosis fetalis. *American Journal of Obstetrics and Gynecology*, 42(6), 925–937. https://doi.org/10.1016/S0002-9378(41)90260-0

Levine, P., & Stetson, R. E. (1939). An Unusual Case of Intra-Group Agglutination. *Vox Sanguinis*, 38(5), 297–300. https://doi.org/10.1111/j.1423-0410.1980.tb02371.x

Stockman, J. A. (2001). Overview of the state of the art of Rh disease: History, current clinical management, and recent progress. *Journal of Pediatric Hematology/Oncology*, 23(6), 385–393. https://doi.org/10.1097/00043426-200108000-00017

Wiener, A. S., & Peters, H. R. (1940). Hemolytic reactions following transfusions of blood of the homologous group, with three cases in which the same agglutinogen was responsible. *Annals of Internal Medicine*, 13(12), 2306–2322. https://doi.org/10.7326/0003-4819-13-12-2306

CHAPTER 3

Alaqeel, A. A. (2019). Hyporegenerative anemia and other complications of rhesus hemolytic disease: to treat or not to treat is the question. *The Pan African Medical Journal*, 32.

Baskett, T. F. (2019). From Tragedy to Triumph: Canadian Connections in the Management of Rhesus Hemolytic Disease of the Newborn. *Journal of obstetrics and gynaecology Canada: JOGC= Journal d'obstetrique et gynecologie du Canada: JOGC*, 41, S207-S214.

Basu, S., Kaur, R., & Kaur, G. (2011). Hemolytic disease of the fetus and newborn: Current trends and perspectives. *Asian journal of transfusion science*, 5(1), 3.

Berentsen, S., & Tjønnfjord, G. E. (2012). Diagnosis and treatment of cold agglutinin mediated autoimmune hemolytic anemia. *Blood reviews*, 26(3), 107-115.

Brojer, E., Husebekk, A., Dębska, M., Uhrynowska, M., Guz, K., Orzińska, A., ... & Maślanka, K. (2016). Fetal/neonatal alloimmune thrombocytopenia: pathogenesis, diagnostics and prevention. *Archivum immunologiae et therapiae experimentalis*, 64(4), 279-290.

Dean, L., & Dean, L. (2005). *Blood groups and red cell antigens* (Vol. 2). Bethesda, Md, USA: NCBI.

Groot, H. E., Villegas Sierra, L. E., Said, M. A., Lipsic, E., Karper, J. C., & van der Harst, P. (2020). Genetically determined ABO blood group and its associations with health and disease. *Arteriosclerosis, thrombosis, and vascular biology*, 40(3), 830-838.

Harman, C. R., Manning, F. A., Bowman, J. M., & Lange, I. R. (1983). Severe Rh disease—Poor outcome is not inevitable. *American Journal of Obstetrics and Gynecology*, 145(7), 823-829.

Hemolytic Disease of the Newborn (HDN). (n.d.). Retrieved from https://www.urmc.rochester.edu/encyclopedia/content.aspx?ContentTypeID=90&ContentID=P02368

Miao, S. Y., Zhou, W., Chen, L., Wang, S., & Liu, X. A. (2014). Influence of ABO blood group and Rhesus factor on breast cancer risk: A meta—analysis of 9665 breast cancer patients and 244 768 controls. *Asia—Pacific Journal of Clinical Oncology, 10*(2), 101-108.

Mollison, P. L., & Cutbush, M. (1951). A method of measuring the severity of a series of cases of hemolytic disease of the newborn. *Blood, 6*(9), 777-788.

Motulsky, A. G., Singer, K., Crosby, W. H., & Smith, V. (1954). The life span of the elliptocyte: Hereditary elliptocytosis and its relationship to other familial hemolytic diseases. *Blood, 9*(1), 57-72.

Noronha, S. A. (2016). Acquired and congenital hemolytic anemia. *Pediatrics in review, 37*(6), 235-246.

Oyelowo, T. (2007). *Mosby's Guide to Women's Health: A Handbook for Health Professionals*. Elsevier Health Sciences.

Pegoraro, V., Urbinati, D., Visser, G. H., Di Renzo, G. C., Zipursky, A., Stotler, B. A., & Spitalnik, S. L. (2020). Hemolytic disease of the fetus and newborn due to Rh (D) incompatibility: A preventable disease that still produces significant morbidity and mortality in children. PloS one, 15(7), e0235807.

Ree, I. M., Smits-Wintjens, V. E., van der Bom, J. G., van Klink, J. M., Oepkes, D., & Lopriore, E. (2017). Neonatal management and outcome in alloimmune hemolytic disease. *Expert review of hematology, 10*(7), 607-616.

Roberts, I. A. (2008). The changing face of haemolytic disease of the newborn. *Early human development, 84*(8), 515-523.

Sarwar, A., & Sridhar, D. C. (2020). Rh-Hemolytic Disease. *StatPearls [Internet]*.

Smits-Wintjens, V. E., Walther, F. J., & Lopriore, E. (2008). Rhesus haemolytic disease of the newborn: Postnatal management, associated morbidity and long-term outcome. In *Seminars in fetal and neonatal Medicine* (Vol. 13, No. 4, pp. 265-271). WB Saunders.

Stanford Children's Health. (n.d.). Retrieved from https://www.stanfordchildrens.org/en/topic/default?id=hemolytic -disease-of-the-newborn-90-P02368

Traut, H. F., & McIvor, B. C. (1946). The Rh factor in obstetrics. *Obstetrical & Gynecological Survey*, 1(3), 350-351.

Weinstein, L. (1982). Irregular antibodies causing hemolytic disease of the newborn: a continuing problem. *Clinical obstetrics and gynecology*, 25(2), 321-332.

CHAPTER 4

Costumbrado, J., Mansour, T., & Ghassemzadeh, S. (2021). Rh Incompatibility. In *StatPearls*. StatPearls Publishing. http://www.ncbi.nlm.nih.gov/books/NBK459353/

Dean, L. (2005). Hemolytic disease of the newborn. In B*lood Groups and Red Cell Antigens [Internet]*. National Center for Biotechnology Information (US). https://www.ncbi.nlm.nih.gov/books/NBK2266/

Infant jaundice—Symptoms and causes. (n.d.-b). Mayo Clinic. Retrieved May 8, 2021, from https://www.mayoclinic.org/diseases-conditions/ infant-jaundice/symptoms-causes/syc-20373865

Iron deficiency anaemia. (2017, October 23). Nhs.Uk. https://www.nhs.uk/conditions/iron-deficiency-anaemia/

Mitra, R., Mishra, N., & Rath, G. P. (2014). Blood groups systems. Indian Journal of Anaesthesia, 58(5), 524–528. https://doi.org/10.4103/0019-5049.144645

Rh Disease—Health Encyclopedia—University of Rochester Medical Center. (n.d.). Retrieved May 5, 2021, from https://www.urmc.rochester.edu/encyclopedia/content.aspx?ContentTypeID=90&ContentID=P02498

Rhesus disease. (2017, October 23). Nhs.Uk. https://www.nhs.uk/conditions/rhesus-disease/

Rhesus disease—Symptoms. (2017, October 23). Nhs.Uk. https://www.nhs.uk/conditions/rhesus-disease/symptoms/

Sarwar, A., & Citla Sridhar, D. (2021). Rh-Hemolytic Disease. In *StatPearls.* StatPearls Publishing. http://www.ncbi.nlm.nih.gov/books/NBK560488/

Vanaparthy, R., & Mahdy, H. (2021). Hydrops Fetalis. In *StatPearls.* StatPearls Publishing. http://www.ncbi.nlm.nih.gov/books/NBK563214/

Westhoff, C. M. (2007). The Structure and Function of the Rh antigen Complex. *Seminars in Hematology, 44*(1), 42–50. https://doi.org/10.1053/j.seminhematol.2006.09.010

Zipursky, A., & Paul, V. K. (2011). The global burden of Rh disease. *Archives of Disease in Childhood—Fetal and Neonatal Edition, 96*(2), F84–F85. https://doi.org/10.1136/adc.2009.181172

CHAPTER 5

Agarwal, K., Rana, A., & Ravi, A. K. (2014, October 9). *Treatment and Prevention of Rh Isoimmunization.* Journal of Fetal Medicine. https://link.springer.com/article/10.1007/s40556-014-0013-z.

Columbia University Irving Medical Center. (2020, August 10). Globally, only half of women get treatment for preventable killer of newborns. *ScienceDaily.* Retrieved May 8, 2021 from www.sciencedaily.com/releases/2020/08/200810113204.htm

Costumbrado, J., Mansour, T., & Ghassemzadeh, S. (2020). Rh Incompatibility. In *StatPearls [Internet].* StatPearls Publishing: Treasure Island (FL).

Dean, L. (2005). Hemolytic disease of the newborn. In *Blood Groups and Red Cell Antigens [Internet]* (pp. 25-30). National Center for Biotechnology Information (US).

Flegel W. A. (2007). The genetics of the Rhesus blood group system. *Blood transfusion = Trasfusione del sangue, 5*(2), 50–57. https://doi.org/10.2450/2007.0011-07

Hamdan, A. H. (2017, July 25). *Pediatric Hydrops Fetalis. Medscape.* https://emedicine.medscape.com/article/974571-overview#a2.

Hamza A. (2019). Kernicterus. *Autopsy & case reports, 9*(1), e2018057. https://doi.org/10.4322/acr.2018.057.

Menkes, J. H., & Curran, J. (1994). Clinical and MR correlates in children with extrapyramidal cerebral palsy. *AJNR. American journal of neuroradiology, 15*(3), 451–457.

Nasser, G. N., & Wehbe, C. (2020). Erythroblastosis Fetalis. In *StatPearls [Internet].*StatPearls Publishing: Treasure Island (FL).

Pegoraro, V., Urbinati, D., Visser, G. H. A., Renzo, G. C. D., Zipursky, A., Stotler, B. A., & Spitalnik, S. L. (2020). *Hemolytic disease of the fetus and newborn due to Rh(D) incompatibility: A preventable disease that still produces significant morbidity and mortality in children.* PLOS ONE. https://journals.plos.org/plosone/article?id=10.1371%2Fjournal.pone.0235807.

Praagh, R. V. (1961, December 1). *Diagnosis of Kernicterus in the Neonatal Period.* American Academy of Pediatrics. https://pediatrics.aappublications.org/content/28/6/870.

Rull V. (2014). The most important application of science: As scientists have to justify research funding with potential social benefits, they may well add education to the list. *EMBO reports, 15*(9), 919–922. https://doi.org/10.15252/embr.201438848

Taylor, M. (2021, March 30). R*h Factor Testing and Pregnancy.* What to Expect. https://www.whattoexpect.com/pregnancy/pregnancy-health/prenatal-testing-rh-factor/.

The Regents of the University of California. (2013). *Fetal Anemia & Thrombocytopenia.* UCSF Fetal Treatment Center. https://fetus.ucsf.edu/fetal-anemia-thrombocytopenia.

Visser, G., Thommesen, T., Renzo, G. C. D., Nassar, A. H., & Spitalnik, S. L. (2020, October 30). *FIGO/ICM guidelines for preventing Rhesus disease: A call to action.* Obstetrics and Gynecology. https://obgyn.onlinelibrary.wiley.com/doi/10.1002/ijgo.13459.

WIRhE. (2020, October 15). *Worldwide Initiative for Rh Disease Eradication.* WIRhE. https://wirhe.org/.

CHAPTER 6

Berg, J. M., Tymoczko, J. L., Stryer, L., & Stryer, L. (2002). *Biochemistry* (5th ed). W.H. Freeman.

Bussel, J. B., & Despotovic, J. M. (2014). Perinatal alloantibody disorders – neonatal alloimmune thrombocytopenia/hemolytic disease of the fetus and newborn. In Reference *Module in Biomedical Sciences* (p. B9780128012383000000). Elsevier. https://doi.org/10.1016/B978-0-12-801238-3.00077-5

Can two Rh-positive parents have an Rh-negative child? (2018, October 9). *Stanford Blood Center*. https://stanfordbloodcenter.org/can-two-rh-positive-parents-have-an-rh-negative-child/

Charles A Janeway, J., Travers, P., Walport, M., & Shlomchik, M. J. (2001). The distribution and functions of immunoglobulin isotypes. Immunobiology: *The Immune System in Health and Disease. 5th Edition.* https://www.ncbi.nlm.nih.gov/books/NBK27162/

Commentary on and reprint of Landsteiner K, Ueber Agglutinationserscheinungen normalen menschlichen Blute [On the agglutination of normal human blood], in Wiener Klinische Wochenschrift (1901) 14:1132–1134. (2000). In Hematology (pp. 769–775). Elsevier. https://doi.org/10.1016/B978-012448510-5.50165-5

Cortey, A., Brossard, Y., Beliard, R., & Bourel, D. (2006). [Prevention of fetomaternal rhesus-D allo-immunization. Perspectives]. *Journal De Gynecologie, Obstetrique Et Biologie De La Reproduction, 35*(1 Suppl), 1S119-111S122.

Dean, L. (2005). *The Rh blood group*. National Center for Biotechnology Information (US). https://www.ncbi.nlm.nih.gov/books/NBK2269/

Fan, J., Lee, B. K., Wikman, A. T., Johansson, S., & Reilly, M. (2014). Associations of Rhesus and non-Rhesus maternal red blood cell allo-immunization with stillbirth and preterm birth. *International Journal of Epidemiology, 43*(4), 1123–1131. https://doi.org/10.1093/ije/dyu079

Flegel, W. A. (2007). The genetics of the Rhesus blood group system. *Blood Transfusion, 5*(2), 50–57. https://doi.org/10.2450/2007.0011-07

Katz, J., Hodder, F. S., Aster, R. S., Bennetts, G. A., & Cairo, M. S. (1984). Neonatal isoimmune thrombocytopenia. The natural course and management and the detection of maternal antibody. *Clinical Pediatrics, 23*(3), 159–162. https://doi.org/10.1177/000992288402300305

Kennedy, G. A., Shaw, R., Just, S., Bryson, G., Battistutta, F., Rowell, J., & Williams, B. (2003). Quantification of feto-maternal haemorrhage (Fmh) by flow cytometry: Anti-fetal haemoglobin labelling potentially underestimates massive FMH in comparison to labelling with anti-D. *Transfusion Medicine (Oxford, England), 13*(1), 25–33. https://doi.org/10.1046/j.1365-3148.2003.00416.x

Krywko, D. M., Yarrarapu, S. N. S., & Shunkwiler, S. M. (2021). Kleihauer betke test. In *StatPearls*. StatPearls Publishing. http://www.ncbi.nlm.nih.gov/books/NBK430876/

Lee, A. I., & Kaufman, R. M. (2011). Transfusion medicine and the pregnant patient. *Hematology/Oncology Clinics of North America, 25*(2), 393–413. https://doi.org/10.1016/j.hoc.2011.02.002

Nester, T. A., Pagano, M. B., & Wu, Y. (2018). Adult transfusion—Principles and practice. In *Transfusion Medicine, Apheresis, and Hemostasis* (pp. 169–200). Elsevier. https://doi.org/10.1016/B978-0-12-803999-1.00008-0

Rh incompatibility | nhlbi, nih. (n.d.). Retrieved May 6, 2021, from https://www.nhlbi.nih.gov/health-topics/rh-incompatibility

Rhesus disease. (2017, October 23). Nhs.Uk. https://www.nhs.uk/conditions/rhesus-disease/

Rho(D) immune globulin monograph for professionals. (2021, April 20). Drugs.Com. https://www.drugs.com/monograph/rho-d-immune-globulin.html

Solomonia, N., Playforth, K., & Reynolds, E. W. (2012). Fetal-maternal hemorrhage: A case and literature review. *AJP Reports*, 2(1), 7–14. https://doi.org/10.1055/s-0031-1296028

The innate and adaptive immune systems. (2020). Institute for Quality and Efficiency in Health Care (IQWiG). https://www.ncbi.nlm.nih.gov/books/NBK279396/

Van Buren, N. (2019). *Transfusion Medicine and Hemostasis* (3rd ed.). https://www.sciencedirect.com/science/article/pii/B9780128137260000507

Wiener, A. S. (1952). History of the rhesus blood types. *Journal of the History of Medicine and Allied Sciences, VII*(4), 369–383. https://doi.org/10.1093/jhmas/VII.4.369

CHAPTER 7

Bhutani, V. K., Zipursky, A., Blencowe, H., Khanna, R., Sgro, M., Ebbesen, F., Bell, J., Mori, R., Slusher, T. M., Fahmy, N., Paul, V. K., Du, L., Okolo, A. A., de Almeida, M.-F., Olusanya, B. O., Kumar, P., Cousens, S., & Lawn, J. E. (2013). Neonatal hyperbilirubinemia and Rhesus disease of the newborn: Incidence and impairment estimates for 2010 at regional and global levels. *Pediatric Research*, 74(S1), 86–100. https://doi.org/10.1038/pr.2013.208

Landsteiner, K., & Wiener, A. S. (1941). STUDIES ON AN AGGLUTI-NOGEN (Rh) IN HUMAN BLOOD REACTING WITH ANTI-RHESUS SERA AND WITH HUMAN ISOANTIBODIES. *The Journal of Experimental Medicine, 74*(4), 309–320.

Stockman, J. A. (2001). Overview of the state of the art of Rh disease: History, current clinical management, and recent progress. *Journal of Pediatric Hematology/Oncology, 23*(6), 385–393. https://doi.org/10.1097/00043426-200108000-00017

Variane, G. F., & Sant'Anna, G. M. (2021). Rhesus disease in Brazil: A multi-professional national survey. *Seminars in Perinatology, 45*(1), 151357. https://doi.org/10.1016/j.semperi.2020.151357

Visser, G. H. A., Thommesen, T., Renzo, G. C. D., Nassar, A. H., & Spitalnik, S. L. (2021). FIGO/ICM guidelines for preventing Rhesus disease: A call to action. *International Journal of Gynecology & Obstetrics, 152*(2), 144–147. https://doi.org/10.1002/ijgo.13459

Winnipeg RH Institute Foundation. (n.d.). Winnipeg RH Institute Foundation. Retrieved May 8, 2021, from https://www.rhinstitutefoundation.org

WIRhE—Worldwide Initiative for Rh Diseas Eradication. (n.d.). Wirhe. Retrieved May 8, 2021, from https://wirhe.org/

CHAPTER 8

Al Dahdah, M., Du Loû, A. D., & Méadel, C. (2015). Mobile health and maternal care: a winning combination for healthcare in the developing world?. *Health Policy and Technology, 4*(3), 225-231.

Balde, M. D., Nasiri, K., Mehrtash, H., Soumah, A. M., Bohren, M. A., Irinyenikan, T. A., Maung, T. M., Thwin, S. S., Aderoba, A. K., Vogel, J. P., Mon, N. O., Bonsaffoh-Adu, K., & Tunçalp, Ö. (2020). Labour companionship and women's experiences of mistreatment during childbirth: results from a multi-country community-based survey. BMJ global health, 5(Suppl 2), e003564.

Bhutani, V. K., Zipursky, A., Blencowe, H., Khanna, R., Sgro, M., Ebbesen, F., Bell, J., Mori, R., Slusher, T. M., Fahmy, N., Paul, V. K., Du, L., Okolo, A. A., de Alemeida, M. F., Olusanya, B. O., Kumar, P., Cousens, S., & Lawn, J. E. (2013). Neonatal hyperbilirubinemia and Rhesus disease of the newborn: incidence and impairment estimates for 2010 at regional and global levels. *Pediatric research*, 74(1), 86-100.

Dela Cruz, R. Z., & Ortega-Dela Cruz, R. A. (2021). Addressing facility management issues and challenges common among public health care institutions in a developing country. *International Journal of Healthcare Management, 14*(1), 107-113.

Human Development Reports. (2020). United Nations Development Programme. Retrieved from http://hdr.undp.org/en/content/human-development-index-hdi

Jung, T., & Harrow, J. (2019). Providing foundations: Philanthropy, global policy and administration. *The Oxford handbook of global policy and transnational administration.*

Lahelma, E. (2001). Health and social stratification. *The Blackwell companion to medical sociology*, 64-93.

Lansang, M. A., & Dennis, R. (2004). Building capacity in health research in the developing world. *Bulletin of the World Health Organization*, 82, 764-770.

Houghton, N., Bascolo, E., & Riego, A. D. (2020). Socioeconomic inequalities in access barriers to seeking health services in four Latin American countries. *Revista Panamericana de Salud Pública, 44*, e11.

Paprotny, D. (2021). Convergence Between Developed and Developing Countries: A Centennial Perspective. *Social indicators research, 153*(1), 193-225.

Pegoraro, V., Urbinati, D., Visser, G. H., Di Renzo, G. C., Zipursky, A., Stotler, B. A., & Spitalnik, S. L. (2020). Hemolytic disease of the fetus and newborn due to Rh (D) incompatibility: A preventable disease that still produces significant morbidity and mortality in children. *PloS one, 15*(7), e0235807.

Shiffman, J., & Smith, S. (2007). Generation of political priority for global health initiatives: a framework and case study of maternal mortality. *The lancet, 370*(9595), 1370-1379.

van der Schoot, C. E., de Haas, M., & Clausen, F. B. (2017). Genotyping to prevent Rh disease: has the time come?. *Current opinion in hematology, 24*(6), 544-550.

Walt, G., & Gilson, L. (1994). Reforming the health sector in developing countries: the central role of policy analysis. *Health policy and planning, 9*(4), 353-370.

Zipursky, A., Bhutani, V. K., & Odame, I. (2018). Rhesus disease: a global prevention strategy. *The Lancet Child & Adolescent Health, 2*(7), 536-542.

CHAPTER 9

Ahmed, R. (2017, June 27). Efficacy of intravenous immunoglobulin in management of rh and abo incompatibility disease - full text view. Retrieved May 07, 2021, from https://clinicaltrials.gov/ct2/show/study/NCT03130517

Cleveland, C. (2018, December 3). Rhesus (RH) Factor. Retrieved May 07, 2021, from https://my.clevelandclinic.org/health/diseases/21053-rh-factor

Costumbrado J, Mansour T, Ghassemzadeh S. Rh Incompatibility. [Updated 2020 Nov 20]. In: StatPearls [Internet]. Treasure Island (FL): StatPearls Publishing; 2021 Jan-. Available from: https://www.ncbi.nlm.nih.gov/books/NBK459353/

Dulay, A. (2020, October). Rh incompatibility (Erythroblastosis Fetalis). Retrieved May 07, 2021, from https://www.merckmanuals.com/en-ca/home/women-s-health-issues/complications-of-pregnancy/rh-incompatibility

Ernst, H. (2018, July 23). Rh Incompatibility. Retrieved May 07, 2021, from https://www.healthline.com/health/rh-incompatibility#effects Erythropoietin. (2011, October). Retrieved May 07, 2021, from https://labtestsonline.org/tests/erythropoietin

Kaneshiro, N., & Zieve, D. (2019, March 6). Rh incompatibility: Medlineplus medical encyclopedia. Retrieved May 07, 2021, from Krywko DM, Yarrarapu SNS, Shunkwiler SM. Kleihauer Betke Test. [Updated 2020 Nov 14]. In: StatPearls [Internet]. Treasure Island (FL): StatPearls Publishing; 2021 Jan-. Available from: https://www.ncbi.nlm.nih.gov/books/NBK430876/

Marshall, S., Husney, A., Romito, K., Gilbert, W., & Jones, K. (2019, May 29). Intrauterine Fetal Blood Transfusion for Rh Disease. Retrieved May 05, 2021, from https://www.healthlinkbc.ca/health-topics/hw149929

Mota M. A. (2013). Red cell and human leukocyte antigen alloimmunization in candidates for renal transplantation: a reality. *Revista brasileira de hematologia e hemoterapia, 35*(3), 160–161. https://doi.org/10.5581/1516-8484.20130046

NHS,—(2018, June 11). Treatment -Rhesus disease. Retrieved May 07, 2021, from https://www.nhs.uk/conditions/rhesus-disease/treatment/#:~:text=During%20phototherapy%2C%20fluids%20will%20usually,need%20for%20a%20blood%20transfusion

Ramasethu, J. (2004). Handbook of pediatric transfusion medicine. In Handbook of pediatric transfusion medicine (pp. 191-208). San Diego, CA, California: Elsevier Academic Press. doi:https://doi.org/10.1016/B978-012348776-6/50021-2

Steinberg, M., & Thein, S. (2021, May 04). Fetal hemoglobin (hemoglobin F) in health and disease. Retrieved May 07, 2021, from https://www.uptodate.com/contents/fetal-hemoglobin-hemoglobin-f-in-health-and-disease

Urbaniak, S. J., & Greiss, M. A. (2000). RhD haemolytic disease of the fetus and the newborn. *Blood reviews, 14*(1), 44-61.

Wagle, S. (2021, April 03). Hemolytic disease of the newborn treatment & management. Retrieved May 07, 2021, from https://emedicine.medscape.com/article/974349-treatment

Wong, R., & Bhutani, V. (2021, February 01). Patient education: Jaundice in newborn infants (Beyond the Basics). Retrieved May 08, 2021, from https://www.uptodate.com/contents/jaundice-in-newborn-inf ants-beyond-the-basics#:~:text=Side%20effects%20%E2%80%94%20 Phototherapy%20is%20very,diapers%20should%20be%20closely%20 monitored.

Yoham AL, Casadesus D. Rho(D) Immune Globulin. [Updated 2020 Nov 30]. In: StatPearls [Internet]. Treasure Island (FL): StatPearls Publishing; 2021 Jan-. Available from: https://www.ncbi.nlm.nih.gov/ books/NBK557884/

CHAPTER 10

Adams, C. (2016, August 21). Why Are There So Many Crazy Theories About Negative Blood Types? *Washington City Paper.* https://washington citypaper.com/article/195000/why-are-there-so-many-crazy-theories-about-negative-blood-types/.

Alonso, S., Flores, C., Cabrera, V., Alonso, A., Martín, P., Albarrán, C., ... & García, O. (2005). The place of the Basques in the European Y-chromosome diversity landscape. European *Journal of Human Genetics, 13*(12), 1293-1302.

Bian, X., Xu, Y., Zhu, L., Gao, P., Liu, X., Liu, S., ... & Wu, Y. (1998). Prevention of maternal-fetal blood group incompatibility with traditional Chinese herbal medicine. *Chinese medical journal, 111*(7), 585-587.

Flegr, J., Hoffmann, R., & Dammann, M. (2015). Worse health status and higher incidence of health disorders in Rhesus negative subjects. *PLoS One, 10*(10), e0141362.

Hullender Rubin, L., Cantor, D., & Marx, B. L. (2013). Recurrent pregnancy loss and traditional Chinese medicine. *Medical acupuncture, 25*(3), 232-237.

Holter, K. (2014). Pregnancy and psalms: Aspects of the healing ministry of a Nigerian prophet. *Old Testament Essays, 27*(2), 428-443.

Hotez, P. J. (2017, February 08). How the Anti-Vaxxers Are Winning. Retrieved from https://www.nytimes.com/2017/02/08/opinion/how-the-anti-vaxxers-are-winning.html

Ilechukwu, S. T. (2007). Ogbanje/abiku and cultural conceptualizations of psychopathology in Nigeria. *Mental Health, Religion and Culture, 10*(3), 239-255.

Kefalew, A., Asfaw, Z., & Kelbessa, E. (2015). Ethnobotany of medicinal plants in Ada'a District, East Shewa Zone of Oromia regional state, Ethiopia. *Journal of ethnobiology and ethnomedicine, 11*(1), 1-28.

Khan, R. (2020). *The Basques May Not Be Who We Think They Are.* Discover Magazine. https://www.discovermagazine.com/the-sciences/the-basques-may-not-be-who-we-think-they-are.

Kilshaw, S., Miller, D., Al Tamimi, H., El-Taher, F., Mohsen, M., Omar, N., ... & Sole, K. (2016). Calm vessels: cultural expectations of pregnant women in Qatar. *Anthropology of the Middle East, 11*(2), 39-59.

Kilshaw, S., Omar, N., Major, S., Mohsen, M., El Taher, F., Al Tamimi, H., ... & Miller, D. (2017). Causal explanations of miscarriage amongst Qataris. *BMC Pregnancy and Childbirth, 17*(1), 1-12.

Lakatos, L. (2004). Bloodless treatment of infants with haemolytic disease. *Archives of Disease in Childhood, 89*(11), 1076–1076. https://doi.org/10.1136/adc.2004.053215

Lezotre, P. L. (2014). State of Play and Review of Major Cooperation Initiatives. *International Cooperation, Convergence and Harmonization of Pharmaceutical Regulations, 7.*

Li, L., Dou, L., Leung, P. C., Chung, T. K. H., & Wang, C. C. (2016). Chinese herbal medicines for unexplained recurrent miscarriage. *Cochrane Database of Systematic Reviews,* (1).

Objectives – Rhesus Solution Initiative. (n.d.). Retrieved from http://rhesussolution.com/index.php/objectives/

Okeke, T., Ocheni, S., Nwagha, U., & Ibegbulam, O. (2012). The prevalence of Rhesus negativity among pregnant women in Enugu, Southeast Nigeria. *Nigerian Journal of Clinical Practice, 15*(4), 400. doi:10.4103/1119-3077.104511

Redfern, N. (2015). *Bloodline of the gods: unravel the mystery in human blood to reveal the aliens among us.* Career Press, Inc.

Sekharappa, V., Amritanand, R., & Venkatesh Krishnan, K. S. D. (2014). Lumbosacral transition vertebra: prevalence and its significance. *Asian spine journal, 8*(1), 51.

Sevilla, S. (2018). Who Built Stonehenge: *The Basque Cro-Magnon.*

Teklehaymanot, T., Giday, M., Medhin, G., & Mekonnen, Y. (2007). Knowledge and use of medicinal plants by people around Debre Libanos monastery in Ethiopia. *Journal of Ethnopharmacology, 111*(2), 271-283.

Tesfaye, S., Belete, A., Engidawork, E., Gedif, T., & Asres, K. (2020). Ethnobotanical study of medicinal plants used by traditional healers to treat cancer-like symptoms in eleven districts, Ethiopia. *Evidence-Based Complementary and Alternative Medicine, 2020.*

Umoh, S. H., & Akinola, T. O. (1994). Nigerian University Students' Awareness of Sickle Cell Anaemia. *Ilorin Journal of Education Faculty of Education University of Ilorin, 53.*

Variane, G. F., & Sant'anna, G. M. (2021). Rhesus disease in Brazil: A multi-professional national survey. *Seminars in Perinatology, 45*(1), 151357. doi:10.1016/j.semperi.2020.151357

Yahia, A., Miskeen, E., Sohail, S. K., Algak, T., & Aljadran, S. (2020). Blood Group Rhesus D-negativity and Awareness Toward Importance of Anti-D Immunoglobulin Among Pregnant Women in Bisha, Saudi Arabia. *Cureus.* doi:10.7759/cureus.7044

Zad, V. R., Khobragade, R., & Saache, S. (2018). Rh-Negative blood: Is It an Alien Blood Group?.

Zipursky, A., Bhutani, V. K., & Odame, I. (2018). Rhesus disease: A global prevention strategy. *The Lancet Child & Adolescent Health, 2*(7), 536-542. doi:10.1016/s2352-4642(18)30071-3

CHAPTER 11

Alsaedi, S. A. (2018). Transcutaneous Bilirubin Measurements Can Be Used to Measure Bilirubin Levels during Phototherapy. *International Journal of Pediatrics*, 2018, e4856390. https://doi.org/10.1155/2018/4856390

Drummond, M., Tarricone, R., & Torbica, A. (2016). Incentivizing Research into the Effectiveness of Medical Devices: Editorial. European Journal of Health Economics, 17(9), 1055–1058.

Hussain, A. S., Shah, M. H., Lakhdir, M., Ariff, S., Demas, S., Qaiser, F., & Ali, S. R. (2017). Effectiveness of transcutaneous bilirubin measurement in managing neonatal jaundice in postnatal ward of a tertiary care hospital in Pakistan. *BMJ Paediatrics Open, 1*(1), e000065. https://doi.org/10.1136/bmjpo-2017-000065

Intramuscular versus intravenous anti-D for preventing Rhesus alloimmunization during pregnancy. (n.d.). https://doi.org/10.1002/14651858.CD007885.pub2

Kaplan, M., Hammerman, C., & Bhutani, V. K. (2015). Parental education and the WHO neonatal G-6-PD screening program: A quarter century later. *Journal of Perinatology, 35*(10), 779–784. https://doi.org/10.1038/jp.2015.77

Pegoraro, V., Urbinati, D., Visser, G. H. A., Renzo, G. C. D., Zipursky, A., Stotler, B. A., & Spitalnik, S. L. (2020). Hemolytic disease of the fetus and newborn due to Rh(D) incompatibility: A preventable disease that still produces significant morbidity and mortality in children. *PLOS ONE, 15*(7), e0235807. https://doi.org/10.1371/journal.pone.0235807

Rai, S., Kaur, S., Hamid, A., & Shobha, P. (2015). Association of Dermal Icterus with Serum Bilirubin in Newborns Weighing <2000 Grams. *International Journal of Scientific Study, 3*(7), 5. https://doi.org/10.17354/ijss/2015/449

Slusher, T. M., Zipursky, A., & Bhutani, V. K. (2011). A Global Need for Affordable Neonatal Jaundice Technologies. *Seminars in Perinatology, 35*(3), 185–191. https://doi.org/10.1053/j.semperi.2011.02.014

* 9 7 8 1 7 7 3 6 9 2 3 9 5 *